Carly Carson

The Truth About Sugar

How Big Name Companies Hide the Truth and the Scientific Facts to Prove It

CRUCIAL TREATS
USA

Contents

Introduction

"I imagine you are feeling a little like Alice now, falling in a rabbit hole?
"You could say that."
"I can see it in your eyes. You have the look of a man who accepts what he sees because he is expecting to wake up. Ironically, this is not too far from the truth. Do you believe in fate, Neo?"
"No."
"Why not?"
"Because I do not like the idea that I am not in control of my life."
"I know exactly what you mean. Let me tell you why you are here. You are here because you know something. What you know, you can't explain. But you feel it. You have felt it your entire life, that there's something wrong with the world. You do not know what it is, but it is there, like a splinter in your mind, driving you mad. It is this feeling that has brought you to me. Do you know what I am talking about?"
"About The Matrix?"
"Do you want to know what it is? The Matrix is everywhere; it is around us, even now, in this very room. You can see it when you look out your window or when you turn on your television. You can feel it when you go to work, when you go to church, when you pay your taxes. It is the world that has been pulled over your eyes to blind you from the truth."
"What truth?"
"That you are a slave, Neo. Like everyone else, you were born into bondage. Into a prison, you cannot taste or see or touch a prison for your

mind. Unfortunately, you cannot tell anyone what the Matrix is about. You must see it for yourself; this is your last chance. After this, there is no turning back: you take the blue pill, the story ends; you wake up in your bed and believe whatever you want to believe. You take the red pill; you stay in Wonderland, and I will show you just how deep the rabbit hole goes."

So now ladies and gentlemen, I don't suppose this short extract is familiar to you, is it?

No, it is not Alice and Wonderland. However, 'the rabbit hole' plays a necessary part in the story I am about to unfold. We will be studying this movie some more. It is the revelatory scene in the Box Office classic when Neo meets Morpheus in the 1990 smash-hit movie *The Matrix* and introduces him to 'the secret.' In *The Matrix*, it 'is everywhere' controlling the world's population under a 'blind [knowledge of] the truth.' In the movie, 'the truth' is that machines control everyone under a computer program that projects a sort of real life. Everyone is living in a dream world, and the real world is a lie. The concept Morpheus opens to Neo is what I want to do with this book, but with another 'secret.'

It is a secret, which has been protecting an equally significant lie, to protect a multi-billion business that governs a whole scale of industries, and what we could call life today. I want to call this a system that I am going to compare to the Matrix. Everyone from the big production companies, especially in alimentation and food production, to the government that we pay high taxes to, but whom also who fund and generate money the business that provides for our health industry. So that when you 'look out your window or turn on your television,' you will see 'the secret' publicized in advertisements. Furthermore, it pays for hundreds upon thousands of jobs and keeps a significant part of the population in 'work.' When consumed in large quantities, it can lead to more severe health issues and conditions to develop over time. So then, it also generates money and business for the health system that you 'pay your taxes' to cover as well. This entire giant infrastructure of industries comes under one governing ingredient, and that ingredient is sugar.

The secret about sugar first appeared on our television screens and media presentations sixty years ago with a sequence of press articles that were released and backed up by governmental bodies, as well as scientific professionals and students. The articles prioritized foods that were high in sugar and protein over eating dietary fat, saying that fat raised cholesterol and could lead to serious health issues, such as obesity, diabetes type 2 and heart disease, among others. One of the first articles to arise was in 1967, when three Harvard students were paid to release their report in *The New England Journal of Medicine,* which minimized sugar's role in developing into heart disease. On the other hand, it hinted towards saturated fats playing a significant role in these negative health issues.

They developed this theory from proclamations instated by American scientist Ancel Keys a decade, or so before with his worldwide study called *the Seven Countries Study*. His research aimed to collect data to prove the adverse effects dietary fat has on cholesterol and heart disease. However, his results were biased and unreliable. Primarily, because he prioritized data from just seven westernized countries, yet there were many other faults to this experiment, which they completely overlooked. We will review it in more detail in chapter two. However, despite the highly invalid evidence he presented to back up his deceiving theory he gained high esteem for his scientific contribution to nutritional advice and became worldwide renowned; however, so did his ideology

I hate to break it to you though; he was wrong, and irretrievably destructive in setting the basis for a fact that set a base for war between fat and sugar! It is a war where most of us have been played like pawns in the middle of a debate, where our health and evolutionary shape are at risk of changing for the very worst. This was only because anyone who tried to contest Ancel Key's theory that fat raised cholesterol was immediately overshadowed and ignored by governing bodies in Scientific Institutions, as well as the government itself. Unfortunately, the businesses go hand in hand as the government funds a large part of the scientific projects and experiments. Furthermore, to publicize your results, they must still meet the criteria of magazines, which the government also checks and funds. They are told what to write, regardless of the evidence being true or not.

Therefore, when they prioritized and favored the publication of these articles, it generated information that forced people to believe contrary to the truth because they read it in a factual magazine like *The Times* or saw it on a scientific documentary. When the media presents us with a message so instructively, our mind naturally registers the facts to be accurate, while we believe it to be backed up by 100% reliable evidence. In general, anything we read or watch on the news we are conditioned to believe is real. As George Orwell once said, *"The people will believe what the media tells them they believe."* It could be all lies for all we know. However, because it is on the news, or stamped with a big, black medical stamp, we will believe everything we see. Furthermore, most of the articles they publicize are under the commanding hand of the government; effectively instill us in following what they inform us to do. Equally for us, as it is for doctors, scientists, teachers, and any Institution that wants to legally function must abide by the law and publish what the government tells them.

However, the big question is: what reason would Institutions and the governments have in lying to us? Why did they go a great extent in spreading this rumor, which then had such detrimental effects on our generation's health and more to come? Why were they so intent on banishing fat from our diet, and replacing it with sugar? In recent decades, nutritionists and biochemists have clarified that sugar is the toxic culprit. Not only this, but it has presented us with health issues that are rocketing sky high with cases in their millions. It is all due to false facts printed in articles and repeated over decades till we became afraid of eating fat. It took such an effect that even to this day we worry about eating too much fat. However, it is all a myth, fat is necessary to our diet, and we should eat all the butter and eggs we can get our hands on!

On the contrary, anything that includes high amounts of sugar, which is just about everything that comes processed and packaged, even a tin of savory baked beans consists of six teaspoons of sugar. We do not realize it is balanced out with salt. That is what we refer to as The Bliss Point Theory, a revolutionary discovery made by Howard Moskowitz, which allowed for the food industry to add as much sugar as possible to drinks, sauces, and all sorts of dietary products. The only trouble is we don't realize how much sugar we are actually eating. On the contrary to stated fact, excess sugar is poisonous to our body and creates adverse effects that, over time, develop into fatal health conditions. The fault is not the fat we eat, which makes us fat either. Although it can get a little confusing considering the name, we have labeled this essential nutrient. It is sugar that causes excess fat to be stored; sugar is the *real* cause of high cholesterol. Therefore, eating, or drinking too much sugar, over time, is a killer!

That is why I am dedicating this book to allowing everyone a chance to find the truth about sugar. I will reveal to you all the answers to the 'secret,' which has purposely been kept undercover for decades. It is a secret that they protected to such an extent that we have witnessed enterprises and governments lying to us publicly via people we entrust with our health and safety, doctors, spokespeople, scientists, journalists, and the rest. However, do not be fooled, thinking the - oh-so 'sweet' and innocent *spice* that we label sugar has been around for only fifty years or a century. The first cultivations of sugar appeared nearly ten thousand years ago in the South Pacific, New Guinea, to be exact. When people began to migrate thousands of years later, they carried sugar with them to other colonies where it drew people instantly to the rich, sweet taste. There it began a journey by passing through India and China to reach Europe and finally to the Americas. It was around the 15th Century, when its journey started to get darker. The little white rabbit has taken us, or should we say 'Alice,' for a leap down the rabbit hole. He's burrowed and burrowed further underground, where the story has only got darker for us till we reach our current position.

Today it stands that 450 million people worldwide have diabetes, and 1.5 billion people are obese. These numbers are expected to escalate in the next twenty to thirty years. It has been projected that in 2050, 95% of people in the USA will be obese. It is all sugar's fault and how it has been implemented in our diet and continues to be reinstated every day through over-advertising. It is even in diet plans, which we believe to be helping us lose weight. Although we have never needed diets, or used them ever before the 1980s, we still wonder why obesity is massively on the rise. However, what we are asking ourselves is; why? How did it get to this stage? Where did 'the secret' begin, and why? Why were we told not to eat fat, but instead to told to eat products fuelled with carbohydrates and sugar? I can imagine you are itching to find out, are you not?

Therefore, let me take you on a journey back up the rabbit hole so that you can see the light and the entirety of the story about sugar. How it began its journey to take complete control of the human race, which is where we stand at this day. So let us go back in time to 8000 BC and the ancient tribes of New Guinea.

The History of Sugar

There is no denying that most of us cannot resist the indulgence of a sweet treat, whether it's a bar of chocolate, a piece of cake, pastry, or a soft fizzy drink. That instant delight that the sweet, sugary taste ignites in us the moment it hits our tongue and runs down our throat, while it sends a signal to our brain that says, 'damn, that's good!' However, damn it, we should, when it triggers that switch in our mind that makes us want more, and more, and more after just one taste. Therefore, making it one of the most addictive drugs on the planet and available in kilos upon kilos lining the shelves of our supermarkets. Not only is it in such high supply, but it feeds a population of extraordinary high scale demand. Unfortunately, some of us do not know how to stop, which has led to the health issues we have today with obesity and diabetes being an enormous pandemic worldwide, especially in the United States.

Reports show that the average American consumes 26 teaspoons of sugar a day, which is the equivalent of 130g of sugar; in a year, it amounts to nearly 50 kilos of sugar. We consume well over a million tons of sugar a year as a collective population. However, sugar was not always in such high supply; it was once a rare commodity. It was all due to industrialization, followed by the invention of high-fructose corn syrup (HFCS). Significantly, that same year the Sugar Federation paid the pioneering Harvard science graduates to write the fraudulent article, which covered up the health issues caused by consuming too much sugar.

However, first I want to take you back in time to share the history of sugar with you, and its journey to the

Americas. These days, you can find sugar in almost everything. In the middle Ages when it first imported into Europe, it was in very short supply. The first cultivation and trading of sugar was organized and pioneered by the Venetians and Cyprians, which made both cities very wealthy at the time. Considering sugar was in such short supply, it was highly sought after by the wealthy and affluent. The high demand for sugar influenced an even higher price tag on it, which meant that it was only accessible by the upper class. Furthermore, it was considered a symbol of status for those who were able to purchase it. Therefore, a new art form appeared in the 14th century where tall, decadent sculptures made of sugar stood up to 6ft tall in the King's hall. You could find the total equivalent of one and a half bags of sugar in the entire United Kingdom. Kings and Queens searched high and wide; they also paid what we would consider to be close $100,000, so they could get their hands on a kilo of sugar. In other words, sugar has always had a substantial green dollar sign above its head, which centuries ago gave it very high value for a minimal amount. Nowadays, it is much cheaper, yet it is mass-produced on a vast scale and consumed equally quickly to ensure it carries on being the most highly traded products in the world, generating billions for the alimentary food industry. However, let us rewind time to see when did the human race get its first taste for sugar?

1.1. THE ORIGIN OF SUGAR

Sugarcane is native to Southeast Asia and the South Pacific. The first sugarcane plants appeared in 8000BC in Papa New Guinea, in the South Pacific. It grew as tall, tropical wild grass that stood up to 20ft tall. The indigenous people of New Guinea would chew on the sweet 'fodder' crop stalks to satisfy themselves between mealtimes, but also used it to fatten up pigs at the start of the agricultural revolution. Although this was a crop recognized in the small island of New Guinea, off the coast of Southeast

Asia, it remained this way for thousands of years. It is important to remember that as humans, our physiology has never depended or evolved on a diet containing refined sugar or carbohydrates. However, in the last 50 years, it has been used in the majority of people's diet plans, which is why we see such adverse effects to our shape, size, and overall health factors. Although it was a crop unknown to the rest of the world, in New Guinea, where it originated, it became legendary. A folk tale told the origins of humankind through a story similar to that of Adam and Eve, considering that the first man and woman sprouted from a sugar cane plant. Therefore, there was no doubt that the enriched flavor had an effect that inspired much thought and passionate debate on its creation and our own. It is a folk take, which linked the appearance of people and sugar in phenomenological philosophy when we began to consider the first religious thoughts. We sought to find a definition of where we came; in other words, a divine creation of God. In Papa New Guinea, they believe we came from sugar. It is not such a silly thought, bearing in mind our primary life source is sugar, just not the same sugar as in sugarcane. We depend on glucose, which is in sugarcane sugar, but mixed with fructose to make sucrose. It is a more concentrated form of sugar, which is why in high supply, it is toxic for us. We make our own sugar, so a highly concentrated additional sugar has adverse effects on our body over time. We will look at this in more detail later.

Sugar began to spread around the South Pacific and Indian Oceans roughly 3500 years ago by the Polynesian seafarers. They carried it over the Pacific, reaching India, where the first record appeared of its organized cultivation in a text that originates from 510 BC. It was when the Emperor Darius of Persia invaded India that he found *the reed which gives honey without bees.* Although the people of India preferred honey, they were the first culture to learn how to chemically refine sugar, and prepare the white sugar crystals we know and love today. The secret spread as far as China, until Emperor Darius transported back to Persia.

One thousand years later, in a twist of fate, the Arabs irreversibly invaded the Persians in 642 AD. They also discovered sugarcane and how to reproduce it for their fructifying benefits. Then, as a result of the Crusades, it reached Europe in the 11th Century, where they first recorded it in England in 1069. When the Crusaders brought back sugar from the Arab *Holy Lands*, they called it 'sweet salt.' However, despite this somehow linear path to Europe, the Ancient Roman and Greek civilizations recorded using it much earlier, in 100 CE, for medicinal reasons. They used it to treat indigestion and stomach ailments.

However, it was not until the Cypriots and Sicilians got their hand on sugarcane with their ideally hot climate and rich fertile soil, which made for perfect conditions in its production. Only then did the real money start to be made with trading sugar, which began in Europe with the Venetians.

1.2. THE FIRST EXPORTATION OF SUGAR

Over 200 years, sugar cane cultivation practices spread from Eastern Europe, mainly Cyprus, to East Africa (Zanzibar). The Lebanese then set up cultivations near Tyre, off the coast of Lebanon. Here, a trade connection was made with Venice, where over time, cultivations moved to Sicily and Venice and overtook the exportation of sugar across greater Europe. None other than the famous merchants of Venice transported it around Europe. Consequently, it made Italy very wealthy and the center point of trade during the 12th Century. Throughout the middle Ages, sugar was a rare commodity and highly sought after in most countries, including England and Spain. People considered sugar a luxury because it came in very short supply and equaled the value of precious gems, such as rubies and diamonds. Furthermore, the Venetians took their opportunity to give it a high price. Therefore, it was purchased only by wealthy people and royalty, or people of high-ranking status.

It was used by the rich as a symbol of status who did not just consume as a sweet condiment. As on thong is for sure, "ordinary people eat food just to sustain themselves, but the wealthy do it to show off." Therefore, sugar was also used as an art material and molded into intricate art sculptures, which would stand ornately, some 6ft tall in the big grand hall. However, no examples remain now dating back to the origin of the art of sugar, drawings and records remain. It was such an expensive commodity that people would tailor into liquid sugar sculptures, a bit like we do with icing sugar on cakes today. Back then, for the rich and famous, 'sugar art' completed the rare decadence that this precious spice portrayed. Once finished, the sugar-icing sculptures would be worth the equivalent of thousands of U.S. dollars in today's money. However, with time they just crumbled to dust and became worthless. One thing was for sure that if people sought so high for sugar and there was money to be made, then the Europeans were going to find a way of exploiting to its full potential. They were in search of new land to cultivate more sugar, as well as faster. It had to be hot with lots of rain; a tropical climate was ideal for growing sugar cane.

Then in the late 1400s, the first large-scale cultivation of sugar cane finally took place in Madeira, organized by the Portuguese. Then around the same time that the Portuguese crossed the Atlantic border to discover South America and landed upon Brazil, they saw the perfect opportunity to cultivate sugar on a grand scale. They established one of the first slave-based plantations here, which then spiraled into a torturous era of the slave trade that started with the production of sugar. At the same time, Christopher Columbus took the idea to cultivate sugar on a large scale in the Caribbean in 1493. In 1540, the Portuguese organized the construction of nearly 3000 sugar cane mills built off the coast of Brazil and another 3000 in the Caribbean in 1550. Here the climate was better than ever before. In the land of the tropical rainforest, sugar was able to grow exceedingly well. It took sugar a few thousand years to leave its place of origin and cross waters. It took just under a hundred years to reach a full-scale worldwide status of cultivation that became the epitome of the darkest moment in the Middle Ages - the Slave Trade. During this time, sugar production laid a black sheet covering the western world with the uncivilized treatment and trade of thousands of Africans used and sold as slaves, which is when our popular sweet spice made its way to America.

So we've seen so far that sugar, although it once grew innocently as a weed in the small island of Papa New Guinea. Once it began its journey across the world, it caused massive uproar. Every pass it inflicted, or was the creation of an invasion or war, until it reached South America first, then influenced the Atlantic slave trade. During the sixteenth and seventeenth centuries, starting with Brazil and the Portuguese who shipped in hundreds of Africans enslaved from North Africa. It was what can be explained as the beginning of mass production and also the New World Order, which they were going to set up in the Americas. They took the opportunity to use the perfectly fertile soil and hot/wet tropical climate off the coast of Brazil, which provided the perfect conditions to cultivate sugar. Therefore, on the island of Santa Catarina, some 2000 mills were constructed to produce sugar on a large scale. Then another 800 mills were built along the north coast of Brazil to supplement more production.

Then the Portuguese moved the farms as far as the Caribbean and built another 3000 mills there too. They shipped in thousands of African men and women to work on the farms. After they discovered Africa in the late 15th Century, they began to trade with African colonies for copper, brass, weapons, and tobacco. They would purchase large quantities of gold, cotton, spices, and people enslaved by their own tribes. The Portuguese placed the slaves to work on the sugar farms that they had set up in Madeira, and then moved them to Brazil, as well as the Caribbean. Finally, all the other countries in Europe caught sight of the immense profits they could make with sugar, so they followed suit, especially as the demand for sugar continued to rise. It fuelled what is seen today as the early colonization times of travel and discovery. Then the Dutch moved their sugar farms into the Caribbean, taking over production in 1658 in the Virgin Islands and Barbados.

Slowly they moved into each of the islands, including Jamaica and Cuba, to construct sugar farms. They also shipped in more and more slaves were across the transatlantic border. Between 1501 and 1587, 12,000,000

Africans were shipped to America and used as slave labor on the sugar, coffee, tobacco and cotton farms. The conditions on the boats that brought them over were so horrific that 25% of them would die on the way, and then endure more sore treatment when they touched down on soil. Sugar was the most popular of the products as everyone consumed it, but also because it fuelled the alcohol business fast on the rise, as well. It made up a fifth of all European imports, where the United Kingdom was considered the highest of its consumers. The Europeans began to invent other condiments such as jam, sauces, chocolates, sweets, and rum. We can see these as the first processed foods and drinks that relied on sugar as its prime ingredient. *"Sugar was something that nobody needed, but everybody craved,"* until its addictive properties, finally made it a necessity. As the production of sugar was much higher by the 16th Century, the price started to decrease. Therefore, it became more accessible to everyone, including the working class. However, this also meant that a higher population of people 'craved' the sweet taste of sugar, so even more sugar had to be produced. However, the soils of the Caribbean isles were starting to get tired.

Therefore, when the British took control of production in Jamaica and Saint Domingue (Haiti) in 1655, they implemented the first irrigation processes, which the French engineers developed, and built irrigation systems, reservoirs, levees, and aqueducts. The innovatory irrigation systems ensured for a better, more fructifying production of sugar. It escalated the production of sugar in such a way that the West Indies produced 80% of sugar exported worldwide. In 1768, the British built the first steam-powered sugar mill factory in Jamaica. It sparked the start of the Industrial Revolution. Then, in the 1740s, Great Britain and The West Indies created *The West India Interest,* where they reaped the large rewards made from the highly profitable business, which sugar production provided. It also gave the British and the French a high status during the colonization of the 17th Century.

During the 18th and 19th centuries, industrialization spread worldwide from the invention of the steam engine in 1712 by Thomas Newcomen, and later developed more efficiently by Jacob Leupold and James Watt. It influenced the development of industries in westernized countries on a large scale. Furthermore, it had a considerable effect on social change during this time, thereby converting us from an agrarian society to an industrialized one. People moved from small villages to cities looking for work in the big factories. Therefore, cities expanded, and an extensive re-organization of the economy for manufacturing took place. However, it had subsequent effects on a worldwide population boom, which fed and demanded mass-production where sugar, amongst many other sugary condiments, could be produced on an even bigger scale than before.

Then in 1747, the German chemist Andreas Marggraf identified that it was possible to obtain sugar from sugar beet plants. They were much cheaper and easier to cultivate, as well as extract the sugar. Furthermore, they did less damage to the soil, which could be seen extensively in the land of the Caribbean from cultivating so much sugarcane. One of his students, Fran Karl Achard, developed his theory and put it into practice in 1789. Achard built his manor and plantation, working alongside King Federick William II of Prussia (Poland). However, Napolean's army burnt it down in 1810 during the Napoleanic Wars, and the French took over its production. Slowly, it took over as the primary form of sugar production, until in 1880 it maximized 50% of exportable sugar, now known as sugar beet.

Further development on the process of extracting sugar via more successful mechanized mediums involved heating sugar using steam, under a partial vacuum. It was invented by the British chemist Edward Charles Howard in 1813. Not only did it save fuel, but it also saved sugar waste lost in the final stage of the sugar refinement process. Then the multiple-effect evaporator developed by the U.S. engineer Norbert Rillieux in the 1820s, made for an even more cost-effective method. Consequently, pioneering American entrepreneurs put these cost-effective processes into practice, building beet factories all over North America. David Lee Child introduced the first beet sugar factory in 1838 to Northampton, Massachusetts.

The first successful commercial sugar beet production took place in California in the 1870s, whereby sugar factories started sprouting up all over North America in significant expansion by the 1890s. From this moment on, sugar production would make North America one of the wealthiest countries on the planet. However, due to its escalated production we see the actual effects that this industrializing change has had on America as it reaches to be the country with the highest rates of Diabetes type 2 and obesity in the world. The reason that you can find sugar in nearly every dietary product available over the counter, even in foods you would never imagine it to be.

1.5. THE FOUNDING OF THE SUGAR FEDERATION

Around the same time that sugar beet factories were appearing all over North America, some of the leaders in the sugar refining industry set up the American Sugar Refining Company (ASRC) in 1889. It helped control the supply and demand for sugar and fixed prices relative to tax, which also ensured that they had a monopolized control over sugar production as well. Therefore, by 1907, the ASRC controlled 97% of all American sugar production.

After that the ASRC formed the Domino Sugar brand at the turn of the Century, in 1900. It operated principally from New York with the Domino Sugar Refinery. Then in 1906, a German immigrant, under the name of David Koncelik, helped form the C& H Sugar (also known as California and Hawaii Sugar Company), which he ran from his sugar beet factory in California. He dominated the production of sugar in both California and Hawaii until the 1930s. The company stayed in existence until 2006, where it was finally bought over by American Sugar Refining (ASR), which was set up in 1998 and instantly started taking over sale production. Today it operates on six separate refineries located in New York, where they took over the creation of Domino Sugar, Maryland, Louisiana, the old C & H refinery in California, Toronto in Canada, and a refinery in Mexico. They have a production capacity of 6.5 million tons of sugar and sweetener products.

In 1942, doctors began warning the public of the health issues related to consuming too much sugar. They advised people to limit the amount of sugar intake as much as possible. Therefore, the government raised the tax on sugar, which inspired manufacturers to turn to the production of high fructose corn syrup (HFCS), also known as glucose-fructose. It is a chemically refined sweetener made from corn starch, which can be grown in an even bigger supply than beetroot or sugar cane. It was first produced in 1967 and is now used to sweeten just about every processed food product on the planet. Although the Food and Drug Administration reiterated, HFCS was safe and harmless to us. They repeated it with the fake articles funded by governmental bodies and the Sugar Association itself.

The Sugar Association was founded in 1943 and has a total of 142,000 members, including growers, processors and refiners of sugar beet and sugar cane, but also man-made sweeteners, such as HFCS.

The in 1967, the Sugar Association's lead executive, John Hickson, commissioned for an article to be released in the *New England Journal of Medicine* by three Harvard scientists to minimize the link between sugar and heart health, forwarding the target at saturated fats. They reinstated this fact, over and over again for over a decade, so that sugar was left unnoticed as having any correlation to heart disease, let alone the full blame. It is not surprising then that in 1968 they became known as the World Sugar Research Organisation, Ltd. (WSRO). No doubt, they instantly wanted to erase this link of fraudulent bribery from their records altogether. Thus, they changed their company name.

Doctors began warning the public from 1942 right up until 1966 of sugar's serious effect on people's health, correlating it to heart disease and Diabetes type 2. However, when the Harvard students released the article in 1967, a war against fat arose. They shunned out the health issues surrounding sugar and began laying the blame on saturated fat. However, this had shocking consequences on everybody's health because *fat* is an essential nutrient that we need to produce natural sugar in our body - glucose. That is right, folks! Our body makes glucose, which we use as fuel to make everything work, from our brain to our muscles, to the general workings of each organ. Therefore, if we add fructose to our body, which is an unknown type to our biological system, then our blood sugar levels rise with it being in excess. An excess of glucose not only builds up as body fat, but raises our cholesterol and heart rate. Therefore, our worldwide epidemic of diabetes and obesity is almost certainly the fault of sugar, not fat. In the next chapter, let us look closer at the series of these catastrophic articles and press releases, which blame fat instead of sugar. For now, I will leave you a recap of the history line displaying how sugar made its journey to the Americas and reached ultimate stardom. At the same time, it molded the world we live in today, both politically and economically.

2

Sugar vs. Fat

It dates back to as far as the 1820s when people first started publishing information that carbohydrates containing starch, as well as sugar, contributed to obesity. Different dietary books included *The Physiology of Taste*, released in 1825, and an important document called *Letter on Corpulence,* written by Sir William Banting in 1864, who was an excessively overweight businessman who weighed 223 pounds, and measured just 5.4 feet. He released his document after being told to eat less sugary products and grain products, including alcohol and more saturated fats and vegetables. Doctors were deliberate in the 1940s to warn people of negative health issues surrounding overeating sugar, saying that it correlated positively with heart disease, amongst other medical conditions that were on the rise after a rise in sugar intake. However, it was nothing to how much we consume today!

Despite the warnings doctors made, few people were aware of them. They had not become very publicly widespread, and few people questioned the health issues anyway. Shortly after the invention of HFCS (High Fructose Corn Syrup), a derivation of grain-based sugar, which is a highly fattening and unhealthy, not considering its chemical process that has its adverse health related to cancer, heart disease, and Alzheimer's disease. The Sugar Association set about protecting their multi-million business to such an extent that they permanently reversed the truth, allowing for tragic results. It was allowed to go on for over 50 years, blinding the greater public from the truth with two complete tools of power, money and the media. The

18

companies implemented in sugar production, including the food companies, restaurants, supermarkets, and all of the other big names in the food industry that make up our daily consumption, thrive off our expenditure on sugar-based products. Why? Because sugar is addictive!

Therefore, to ensure this absolute empire that sugar had become after centuries of working its way to the top. There was no doubt that they were going to allow it to disappear off the shelves that quickly. However, to do this, they would have to reverse the truth and fast. Society in our modern world, since industrialization, acts much faster mainly to cover a myth. That is because news travels so much quicker today with advanced technology and the media. Where in the 1400s, we might have taken some 50 to 100 years to act and develop an idea. Then pre-BC, it could take up to a millennia to react. It took over 5000 years for us to discover sugar where only the indigenous tribes of New Guinea indulged in this rare sweetener. It then took another 2000 years for it to travel across the world and finally reach Europe, then another 600 years before it was properly introduced to America. All this time and for hundreds of thousands of years, we survived mainly off the natural animal and plant-based products relying heavily on their vitamins and nutrients, as well as protein and saturated fats. However, people now acted fast. They had created a dangerous yet highly profitable formula like that of HFCS, which would be on sale in plain sight for everyone to consume at their leisure, a guilty pleasure that had to remain unseen. It meant they would have to completely reverse the truth on dietary health, which they did; a year later.

A classic case of conspiracy fraud, which was funded by none other than the Sugar Federation to ensure they could continue supplying their toxic drug at an extensive rate, in as many products as possible. They paid a group of Harvard science students to backup and certify that saturated fats were associated with weight gain and heart disease. The information led the public's eye away from the destructive effects of sugar and cut saturated fats like butter, eggs, or fatty meat out of people's diet. The theory Ancel Keys had shed light on in the 1950s, they kept forcing into the public eye right up until the 1980s. In documentation released recently, it reveals the truth, and the horrific measures taken to prevent this fatal secret from reaching the public eye. It is this apparent truth, which is set before our eyes every day to show us why obesity has risen out of control, and consequently, diabetes as well. Do you think saturated fats were at fault, which is why we were told to cut them out of our diet? So why have we seen cases in these two human-made diseases reach numbers like never before? The numbers are rising out of control, especially in the United States, and they do not seem to be slowing down.

The fault lies within a complex web of lies, to which I am going to reveal to you in this chapter, so sit tight and prepare yourselves for what you are about to hear is not pretty, it's almost unbelievable, but believe me it is 100% true!

2.1. FIRST WARNINGS SUGAR AFFECTS OUR HEALTH

Now then, before we start to look at the fraudulent cases that changed our beliefs on dietary nutrition for the worst. Let us go back to the turn of the 19th Century when sugar and carbohydrates first became accessible to the greater public. Until the Age of Industrialization, these supplement ingredients had been a luxury in high demand. However, supply had risen extensively out of the expansion from cultivating sugar in new, more fertile land in the Americas. The cheap labor provided by the transatlantic slave trade accelerated business potential even more. However, it also left a dark shadow of poverty, suffering, and uncivilized behavior, which the white-Caucasian Europeans and North Americans inflicted upon the Africans. On the transatlantic journey, from Africa to America, the conditions on the ships were so awful that only three-quarters of the slaves on board made it to the other side. Upon their arrival on shore, it was merely a fight for survival to anyone who was to begin working on the crop fields, cultivating sugar amongst other products in high demand and production.

Finally, by 1804, all U.S. states had abolished slavery, although racism and prejudice towards the Africans continued for much longer. However, steam-powered engines and machines, as well as more cost-effective mass production processes, were discovered. Therefore, sugar production continued to an ever-rising state until it reached a state of excess in demand. As more people were able to indulge in its tastes, it no longer became a luxury, but a necessity. We did not necessarily need a condiment in our diet, but one we desired more than any other. It could be in the form of an alcoholic beverage, which is merely fructose-sugar fermented, or it could be a tasty sweet treat like a cake, pastry, chocolate bar or sweets. However, when it was accessible to everyone and available in high supply, the secondary effects in people's health began to show. In the early days, as it was a new dietary ingredient to our usual daily menu. It was evident that anything out of the ordinary that appeared in someone's health factors was likely to be a consequence of this unfamiliar food we had begun to supplement in our diet.

The first record of information publicized about the harmful effects of sugar on our body appeared in the 1820s. However, during the Tudor Times in Britain, you could see in the iconic figure of the over-sized King Henry VIII who famously re-married seven times, abolishing the Catholic Church in Britain, and horrifically beheading two wives including Anne Boleyn. Unfortunately, diet was not a subject of study in his day. However, what we are aware of, is that the upper class and royalty especially; suffered from malnutrition. In the cities, there was a sewage and irrigation problem. Therefore clean water was in short supply. Instead, they opted for alcohol where they drank beer and wine by the gallon. This sugar-fermented drink can have adverse effects on someone's health, as well as mood swings. Then vegetables were considered to be a food eaten by poor people. Therefore, the rich and wealthy lived off a diet of meat, bread, wine, beer, and sweets. It is no reason their life expectancy depreciated excessively during this time. Now, let us look in more detail at the two documented records, which appeared in the 1800s, focusing on our susceptibility to malnutrition. It all started in France, the capital of Gastronomy! During this time, the French were experimenting and studying food like no other nation. One such man was Jean Anthelme Brillat-Savarin, a French lawyer and gourmet fanatic, and began researching into the subject of diets as early as 1825. He then released his first book on nutrition in 1863 called *The Physiology of Taste*, which concluded his observation that the same thing they fed to fatten up livestock (pigs, cows, and sheep) would have the same effect on humans; it will fatten them up. Around the same time in London, England, a man named Sir. William Banting, who was of short stature standing at 5.4 feet tall, happened to weigh an excessive 223 pounds. He attempted a variety of different ways to lose weight until he met a doctor who had studied in France. He recommended Sir. William should drink less alcohol, as well as eat less sugary products and grains. Instead, he should focus only on a diet that consisted of meat, fish, cheese, and vegetables, and after doing just this in less than nine months, Sir. William lost 40 pounds of excess weight. He went on to publicize the revelatory advice the doctor gave him on dietary nutrition in a paper called *Letter on Corpulence*, which he released in 1864. Such advice continued into the 20th century when people asked about their nutritional health. However, it was quite infrequent because other epidemics were taking place at the start of the 20th Century, namely World War I and II. The rationing during this time meant that health was not very affected by sugar because most people were not allowed to eat much of it anyway. However, in the 1940s, health specialists observed that the highest death rate in the U.S. was due to coronary disease. Doctors reiterated the adverse effects of sugar on people's health, correlating heart disease to an excess of sugar intake. Most medical institutions actively gave counsel to their patients, advising them to consume as little sugar as possible – right up until 1966. However, coronary disease was not just an effect of eating excessive amounts of sugar, but it was also due to smoking. Tobacco and smoking was a habit that had become the norm in most men and women during the 1930s and 40s. Therefore, it would have also had a significant effect on the results, proving heart disease to be America's biggest killer.

The raised skepticism over the health issues related to sugar at this time, which included heart disease, saw the rise of the artificial sweetener industry. Firstly, they invented calcium cyclamate, which appeared in sodas and fizzy drinks in 1952. However, the food industry banned it shortly after because they discovered it to be carcinogenic. Then they made Aspartame (NutraSweet) in 1965, which they also removed quickly. However, when they finally found high fructose corn syrup (HFCS) in 1967, the Sugar

Association took great care, ensuring it was safe for consumption. Recent studies have proven otherwise. You produce high fructose corn syrup from corn starch by breaking down the glucose enzymes, and supplementing fructose through a process of heating with hydrochloric acid. The method of making HFCS proved extremely cost-effective and much easier to handle than ordinary beet sugar production. The good thing about corn is that it can grow anywhere in high volume, and fast. Therefore, in the 1970s companies like the Clinton Corn Processing Company and the Japanese Agency of Industrial Science came into practice producing gallons of the syrup. Slowly but surely, it became implemented in all processed foods, which had adverse effects on people's health. We are going to look at this in more detail in chapter: *The Rise of the Artificial Sweetener.*

Until the 1960s, they were still enlightening us into the truth and warning us about the effects that our guilty pleasure for sweets – had on our health! Then, Ancel Keys objected to this fact in the late fifties, and continued to do so till the mid-seventies. He was the first figure of scientific authority to start correlating saturated fats, high in cholesterol, as having detrimental effects on our health, especially heart disease. In other words, he proposed that the food our diet has depended on for hundreds of thousands of years, one of which food types is saturated fat, is bad for us. He proposed that instead, we should eat more sugar and grain, which we had always used to fatten up livestock, and guess what? we believed him! What I want to look into is why?

First of all, it was because we had never really considered what it is that we had to eat. We have been so busy reacting to the world that is always changing around us. Therefore, what goes on inside of us doesn't matter to us. However, there are other factors, as well. First of all, we were supplied this information by believable parties. These include the media, scientists, pediatrics, and nutritionists. We are reliant and expectant of them to provide the information correctly, so we believe them. Anything they say, we will accept. When the message is repeated to us excessively over time, then even if it is just decades, for us, it is a lifetime. It then becomes imprinted entirely in our cognitive beliefs. Any other information before this will be out of the ordinary and unfamiliar, so we may choose not to believe it. It happened in

1972, when John Yudkin attempted to speak out at these revelations, which were being made by Ancel Keys and the three Harvard students who released their article in 1967. However, they had Yudkin immediately eliminated from the scene, and his debate and writings, which he published with information contrary to the advisors, such as Ancel Keys, who were backed up by the institutions – were quickly taken off the shelves.

Any advice that was contrary to that made be Ancel Keys in the 1970s was ignored. He had the agreement and defense of the Institutions in Science, as well as the government. Therefore, he had the first word, whether it was wrong or not. Again and again, this hierarchical, unjust behavior took place throughout the 70s and 80s. Therefore, allowing for a giant carpet to cover the truth comfortably setting station for a mass-market of sugar consumption by the metric ton, on a day-to-day basis. Large corporate companies took advantage of this secrecy and actively sponsored the implementation of sugar in nearly every food product available. The rise of the processed food industry began, which included the highly concentrated, but carcinogenic artificial food sweetener – high fructose corn syrup (HFCS). It is present in 99% of processed foods and drinks, such as ketchup, sodas, ready-made meals, and many, many more. It proved to be an extremely profitable ingredient, especially with the 'Bliss point' theory discovered by Dr. Howard Moskowitz in the 70s, meaning that companies could add as much HFCS as they liked, by balancing out the sweet taste with salt. In some products like soda drinks, you can find the equivalent of up to 10 teaspoons of sugar – in just one serving! However, it has also had adverse effects on our health. After all, it drives inflammation and the build-up of body fat by increasing our triglyceride levels.

2.2. COUNTING CALORIES

Now before we turn to the war against saturated fats and sugar, where scientists and governing bodies began to shift the public eye from believing that sugar was bad for you to fat, I want to take a quick look at the studies, which they did on calories. The development of calories is vital in the whole dietary scheme of things because it was the final link that allowed people to ignore the toxic effects of sugar completely, and become obsessed with their weight by cutting fat out of their diet. The reason for this was when we started to measure our food allowance in calories, first applied in one of the first books on dieting written by an American writer called Lulu Hunt Peters.

In 1918, Lulu H. Peters wrote *Diet and Health (with the keys to calories)* where she proposed the first concept of counting calories as a way of regulating weight control. However, Peters took her inspiration from an experiment carried out by an American chemist called Wilbur Olin Atwater in the 1880s, which also lacked viability. Although it was an interesting theory for its time, it probably needed further research. Wilbur Olin Atwater studied the work of a French engineer named Nicolas Clement-Desormes. In the 1820s, Nicolas Clement-Desormes first used the word 'calorie' to describe the unit of energy so he could distinguish the capacity of different motor engines.

Atwater used this metric terminology and idea to distinguish the capacity of energy released when he burnt different food groups like carbohydrates, fats, legumes, etc. He found that fat burned double the amount of 'calories' to carbohydrates. In other words, the fat burnt off around nine calories, where the carbs just burnt off four calories.

However, in 1918 when Lulu H. Peters included this theory as the basis for her best/selling book, it was still very early days to start making any presumptions on metric energy distinguishing different food types. For one thing, Atwater turned a philosophy, which Nicolas Clement-Desormes used to compare engine fuel - as a comparison for a person's diet. In other words, Atwater compared a human's body to a 'car engine.' Additionally, Peters had little knowledge and understanding of science. She did not have the medical qualifications or expertise to write about dieting and nutrition the way she did, but also receive as much praise and attention.

In fact, most of us still swear by her ideology, as well as Ancel Keys. He developed the idea one step further, and both these figures soared to stardom by publishing false information that would change the history of humankind forever. *Diet and Health (with the keys to calories)* hit the top seller mark in 1922, and it didn't lift till 1926! She prophesized that our weight depended on how many calories we ate in a day. The more calories we eat, then the more weight we put on. Her theory advised that the average person should eat 1500-2000 calories a day, the exact amount depended on our age and height, which became widely known as our BMI (Body Mass Index). Peters theorized that if someone exceeded this limit, then they would have to work off the calories to keep a healthy weight and size. Most of today's dietary and nutritional advice still follows Peters' theory on calories. A few essential points were left out. Firstly, both Peters and Atwater considered all food types to be the same. In other words, 100 calories of carbohydrates are equal to 100 calories of fats, which is also equal to 100 calories of vitamins. Do you think that is a fair comparison? I would like to argue this fact because 100 calories of carbohydrates does not provide the same nutrition as vitamins and fats, even though they might have the same calories. Furthermore, each food type burns differently in our body. Fat, for example, burns much quicker and provides more nutrition than carbohydrates, which give very little. Secondly, everyone's body is different. We all have a different metabolic rate, which is our system of breaking down food and burning it off as energy as glucose. Therefore, how did we got to measuring our diet in calories when all food types are different, and all body types are different too. Peter's book on dietary advice, *Diet and Health (with the keys to calories),* was one of a kind. It was also ahead of its time when she published it in the 1920s. It gave preliminary insight into dieting and nutrition, yet unfortunately, no one developed the theory any further. Unfortunately, they did not do this in the right way. The facts Lulu H. Peters suggested lacked reliable evidence and further study for future specialists to rely so heavily on them, as a reference for dieting. Then again, we are about to meet her partner in crime, who was Ancel Keys. He also got too much credit for spreading a false truth, which everyone believed again.

2.3. 'THE FRAUD OF THE CENTURY'- ANCEL KEYS

Ancel Keys (1904 - 2004) was an American Physiologist. He had a long life and an even more successful career. During World War II, he established himself as a physiologist and contributed a lot to the soldiers' military diet regime. He created what was known as the K-ration, which allowed for a soldier to eat foods in short supply while filling up on 3200 calories, necessary to keep them alert and active in battle. To further his study on wartime nutrition, he carried out an unethical experiment in 1944, called the Minnesota Starvation Experiment, where he inflicted a series of fasting programs on 32 subjects.

In some cases, groups would undergo intensive stages of not eating to test the mental and physical effects that starvation can do to the human body. It was not until 1950 when Ancel Keys, accompanied by his wife, traveled the world and carried out their famous, yet ruinously inaccurate scientific research called *The Seven Countries Study*. They wished to explore the effects that different foods have on our health factors, mainly the risk of heart disease as it remained the leading cause of death in America.

Keys extensive research lasted nearly 20 years. His first set of findings he published in 1958, then he finally finished his lengthy study in 1970, testing a total of 12,770 men. Although he collected data in many more countries, he only released the findings of seven particular ones. In a world with over 180 countries, Keys felt that only seven were sufficient representatives of a worldwide study. He missed out on all the countries where the results didn't match up, which were most of them. His experimental thesis proposed that cardiovascular disease (CVD) was directly correlated to high cholesterol in the blood, which happens when we eat too many saturated fats. North America had the highest rates of heart disease worldwide, and they also ate the most fat. Japan recorded the least amount of deaths with the least amount of fat intake. Whereas, Italy had the highest number of people aged over 80 and lived on a strict carbohydrate diet, eating pizza and pasta. On this over-simplified observation, he set the grounds for one of the most significant misinterpretations of scientific data in history. Many scientists who believed contrary to him tagged as - 'The Fraud of the Century,' such as George Mann. However, one thing that Ancel Keys did not include in his findings was 'sweets'; neither did he include smoking. Therefore, just how accurate were the results, when the two most probable causes of cardiovascular disease were missing. Despite these unreliable results, he received many rewards and esteemed acknowledgment for this false proclamation that was to have a more severe effect on our society's health than was ever envisioned. All we wonder is – why?

Ancel Keys had already established a high position in his early career by working his way up the ladder in the scientific institutions funded by government jobs during World War II. He was responsible for the K-ration diet, followed by military soldiers in WWII, which balanced their diet into calories. He used Peters' theory on the average daily calorie of 2000 calories for the average man, and upped it to 3500 for the intensive combat and fasting they might have had to endure in battle. Therefore, the Institution quickly accepted his theory that saturated fats raised cholesterol and worsened the risk of heart disease. He received extra credit in 1955 when the American President in power, Dwight D. Eisenhower, suffered a severe heart attack. On the very next day, Sir Eisenhower's physician, Dr. Paul White, gave a famous press conference that defended Key's lipid hypothesis. Firstly, he advised people to stop smoking and reduce stress to prevent the onset of a heart attack. However, he also recommended that people should reduce saturated fat and cholesterol as well.

Then on January 13, 1961, Keys appeared on the front cover of *The Times* magazine, which was one of the most prestigious magazines in the U.S. The headlines read: *"Diet and Health,"* where he talked passionately about his theory, which he became renowned forever. It was that *'fat raises cholesterol, and it is responsible for heart attacks.'* That same year, the American Heart Association (AHA) and the National Institute of Health (NIH) also began recommending to people to avoid fat and cholesterol. That same year and after six years of investigation, Dr. Kannel and Dr. Dawber published their results from the *Framingham Heart Study*. They concluded that total cholesterol is a reliable indicator of heart attacks. In other words, they found that if you have high cholesterol, you will most likely have a heart attack. The *Framingham Heart Study* is one of the most extensive, crucial epidemiological studies in medical history. In the 1960s, it helped fuel one of the first anti-smoking campaigns for the data, which specialists collected correlating it to heart disease. However, for its official status, then any information linked to heart disease, for example, Kannel and Dawber relating it to saturated fats – well, we believed them!

So, from this moment on, the Institutions and the U.S. government told doctors to advise people to reduce saturated fat in their diet. It also paved the perfect opportunity for the Sugar Association to reiterate this statement conclusively. They took the theory proposed by Ancel Keys that saturated fats were bad for us one step further. However, this time they bribed a group of students to defend Ancel Keys' theory and divert the public eye entirely away from sugar as much potential, let alone - absolute culprit! The fact remained, and although brave biochemists and nutritionists attempted to attack it, they only risked losing their careers and livelihoods objecting to Key's dangerously, inaccurate theory. No one could rival his popularity and power in the Institutions of Science, as well as the government and media. He was the celebrity of science throughout the 60s and 70s. He was also the only scientist to receive so much credit in his time, appearing on the cover of *The Times* magazine. However, his theory was so wrong. Saturated fats aren't bad for the heart. Instead, your heart needs them to stay healthy. On the other hand, sugar is bad for your heart. However, what you are about to find out will test that theory forever. Unfortunately, the entire human race was going to be in the middle and affected by it. It is why heart disease has reached exceeding numbers. However, it is not because of smoking because these numbers have gone down in recent decades, but because of excess consumption of sugar.

2.4.THE CASE AGAINST FAT CONTINUES

So now that Ancel Keys did his part in the mechanical network of dietary lies, which were the center of the public's attention in the late sixties. However, medical professionals were still recommending people in some areas that sugar was also related to diabetes and cardiovascular disease. Therefore, companies associated with the Sugar Association began making artificial sweeteners as a way of disguising sugar in food, especially in soda drinks. However, the Food Federation caught them out by banning each sweetener until they came up with high fructose corn syrup (HFCS). HFCS was allowed and proved a more cost-effective formula, as well as a higher concentration of glucose-sugar. However, it was also highly carcinogenic, even more so than sugar beet.

Although the Sugar Association took a big risk, they were also very intent in protecting their multi-million empire that had taken centuries to develop and maintain. Even in the 1960s, hundreds of businesses and employees were at a risk of losing their jobs if people stopped consuming sugar. They had to be ahead of the game! They realized that scientists and the media had a lot of influence on people's way of thinking and perceptions. As the famous science-fiction novelist George Orwell once said, *"The people will believe what the media tells them they believe."* Although we would like to think otherwise, he is right. When we see something on the news - nine times out of ten, we will believe it because of the media is presenting the information in an alerted way. Your brain instantly registers the information as reliable if it comes from a scientist's voice, and primarily via an established factual magazine or an academic seminar. It is the very way they project the information to us that we have no choice to believe it is undeniably true.

In 1967, a group of Harvard science graduates wrote an article, which they released in the *New England Journal of Medicine*. The article minimized the adverse effects of sugar on cardiovascular disease (CVD), and instead shifted the blame to saturated fats. It built on the hypothesis made by Ancel Keys, which the U.S. President Dwight D. Eisenhower approved in 1955

when he suffered a heart attack and diagnosed with cardiovascular disease.
The Association paid the Harvard students to print false information taking
the pressure off the real culprit of cardiovascular disease, other than
smoking - sugar. However, who would have known that the Sugar
Association was the original funders for this press release. They paid each
student what the equivalent of today's money - $50,000, so they rereleased
proclamations forwarding the fault to fat. Thus, allowing the food industries
to continue in business unseen by the public eye, producing sugar on an
immense scale. It didn't stop here either. After receiving a large amount of
backlash cases from scientists who were more intuitive and outspoken to
this utter false myth, they had to reinstate the fact a little more.

On March 26th, 1984, *The Times* magazine released an edition where the
front cover depicted a sad face with a slice of bacon turned down and two
fried eggs for eyes. It was commissioned by none other than Senator George
McGovern, who was following a strict vegan diet and did not eat meat or
derivations, such as eggs, butter, etc. Therefore, when the headlines read in
big yellow capital letters, "Cholesterol is deadly," it was the final turn of the
knife that completely reversed our impression of a diet we had depended on
for millennia. It paved the way for what was to promote a low-fat diet when
doctors counseled people on losing weight. However, this ignorance of the
truth wasn't just slightly inefficient; it was devastating for our modern-day
health on a global scale. Even when people wanted to try and lose weight,
they could not because they were being given the wrong advice. It is why
we have seen obesity soar out of the roof, despite the effort being made to
come up with different diets. None of them work because they are all based
on the false ideology that fat is the reason we have excess fat, just because it
is in the name – we have believed them. Well, we couldn't have been more
wrong, could we!

2.5. SUGAR IS PURE, WHITE AND DEADLY (JOHN YUDKIN)

Professor John Yudkin was a physiologist and nutritionist who dedicated his career from the 1950s onwards, professing the very opposite to Ancel Keys' theory, which correlated fat to coronary disease. Instead, Yudkin advised people to follow low-carbohydrate diets to lose weight. In 1972, he published a book called *Pure, White and Deadly* in the U.K., which they released as *Sweet and Dangerous* in the U.S. The title printed in the United States was considerably less aggressive than the U.K. version. He had it translated in eight languages only, which did not include French and Spanish. It warned people of the dangers sugar proposed to our health, including CVD, as well as dental healthcare problems like cavities, diabetes, liver disease, cancer; the list goes on…

However, Yudkin did not succeed in taking the limelight off Ancel Keys or the theory that was to blame for malnutrition health issues. His arguments were not backed up by the Institutions or the governing authority. On the hand, Ancel Keys was. Therefore, when Keys denounced Yudkin's theory that sugar was at the 'heart' of the problem, Yudkin did not have a 'leg to stand on.' A fragment of Keys' critique included that:

"It is clear that Yudkin has no theoretical basis or experimental evidence to support his claim for a major influence of dietary sucrose in the etiology of CHD & and his "evidence" from population statistics and time trends will not bear up under the most elementary critical examination."

Ancel Keys had received a lot of acclaim in his career by the parties in control of the magazine publications and Institutional scientific organizations, and his word won over Yudkin's. Therefore, shortly after John Yudkin made his acclaim, then his books soon disappeared off the shelves. His career reached a cold, fast finish with little approval until the 21st-century hit, where Robert Lustig had his say and fortunately with success. However, first American biochemist George Mann, in 1991, released his results that clearly showed:

For every 1% mg/dl lowered cholesterol, 11% of deaths increased due to heart disease.

Mann's theory not only testified that of Ancel Key. It also hypothesized that if we don't eat fat, it raises our risk of heart disease, not the other way round. Mann went on to say that Ancel Keys was "the major scientific fraud of the century, and maybe of any century." That same year, William P. Castelli, director of the *Framingham's heart study* (an ongoing investigation since 1948- into the research of the causes of CVD) wrote: "the more saturated fat is consumed, lower is the cholesterol, and lower is a person's body weight." However, Mann's revelatory conclusion was not publicized to such an effect as it should have been, unlike Keys theory that saw him rise to fame in the 70s. However, we ask ourselves why this was so?

Robert Lustig managed to reach a much larger audience in 2009 with his video presentation, where he linked the fructose component of sucrose (sugar) to the development of the metabolic syndrome, which in effect led to severe health issues, including Diabetes type-2, coronary disease, liver disease and obesity. He declared passionately, "which was worse the sugar or the fat, the sugar a thousand times over!" He believes that our diet was altered and adulterated under our sight over the past fifty years to keep the food industry productive using sugar as their main lethal ingredient. He saw "fat go down" as a result of what fraudulent scientists, such as Ancel Keys had said to defend the Sugar Association, and gain fame and fortune. Consequently, he "saw sugar go up," and also saw how, "we're all getting sick."

Why? Sugar is toxic.

He went on to praise scientists, such as John Yudkin, for their attempt to spread the truth. However, he also professes at their unjust treatment, and eventual career failure due because of the reputation wrongly spread about them to defend the system's mechanical network of lies.

We wonder how Robert Ludwig was able to voice this controversial message in light of everything said. Fortunately, he made his fame on YouTube, which has proven to be an excellent method for spreading information via media videos shared on this popular internet web platform. Since they launched the website in 2005, it has become a popular tool of entertainment and is watched and used by billions. Therefore, it is an excellent tool for marketing and rising to fame quickly and much more easily. It opened up a whole new talent of people who once had to pass through hierarchical mediators that control the music industry from the top—a bit like in the science world. Therefore, not every amazing talent reaches the public eye. Ed Sheeran is one such multi-million artist who found fame on YouTube. Then there is a whole industry of kid-stars who have made their fame via this excellent media tool, who are great at advertising kids' games and toys. They are also watched by millions of children worldwide, especially nowadays. YouTube has allowed for information on taboo subjects that were once kept secret from us - finally be revealed. One such video was this made by Robert Lustig, and quite rightly, he shot to fame for the right reasons allowing for his revelatory message to be shared and reached by more, which gave him the credit that he may not have been granted. It also enlightens us into another issue, just how much should we believe – that we see on the news?

3
What is Sugar?

Sugar is the generic name for sucrose. It is a pure and soluble form of carbohydrate made up of sucrose and glucose. Therefore, when you digest sugar, it instantly produces a chemical reaction in our body, which fuels us with energy. The energy keeps the general mechanisms of our body working throughout the day, whether it is to feed our muscles, our brain, or to keep our digestive system regularly working to effect. Therefore you would imagine sugar to be essential to our diet, wouldn't you? Well, maybe it is at times. Although, most of us do not actually need it unless we live very active lives, which most of us do not in this modern day. We use public transport or cars to move around, and we are dependent on technology and electro-domestic appliances that have made our daily living much more comfortable, but also less demanding of our time and physical activity. The only people nutritionists advise these days correctly to up their carbohydrates and glucose levels are sportspeople. People who are active, or take part in sports, are regularly burning off energy throughout the day. Therefore, they require extra supplies of glucose and carbohydrates to maintain their active lifestyle, providing them additional stores of energy fuel.

The fact is, our body is already designed to make this fuel, which is glucose. Your digestive system is an active processor, which produces it naturally, in your liver. The pancreas also works to regulate the blood sugar levels by secreting a hormone called insulin. Therefore, when we supplement our body with more sugar in the form of fructose, or even sucrose, we are upping our sugar levels with excess sugar. There are different types of sugar. First of all, there is glucose, which is the sugar produced widely by the mammal animal group type. Then there is fructose, which is present in plant-based products, such as fruit and vegetables. Sugarcane and sugar beet are the two vegetables classed as having the highest concentration of fructose. Then in the refining of sugarcane and sugar beet, a process adds glucose to make sucrose. Sucrose is the sugar we know today in the pure white crystals, or even brown and golden. The color of the sugar depends on what stage of the refinement they have been stopped. Brown sugar is produced just after it has crystalized when it has caramelized and dried. Therefore, it still contains some of the molasses coating, which gives it a slightly bitter-sweet taste. Sucrose is also present and naturally made in lactose products, such as milk, yogurt, and other dairy items.

Sucrose sugar is something people have always craved, and also loved. Once upon a time, we searched high and wide for just one bag of sugar – we would pay tens of thousands of dollars for it. Even to this day, we see a sweet treat, and we just can't resist. We get a reward from eating it because it tastes good. That is because sugar is highly addictive. We eat one sugary snack, and we want one after another, after the other. However, this is dangerous to our health despite the false statements made by doctors and scientists of the late 20th century. Sugar is very bad for us. It is shown today in the high numbers of people who suffer from different illnesses now associated with sugar. These include diabetes, obesity, liver disease, heart disease, Alzheimer's disease, and more.

It is essential to know what it is we are eating, as well as what is healthy and what is not. Over-consumption of sugar, which occurs every day by three-quarters of the world population, is very toxic to our body. It has produced millions of cases of adverse health issues, which are set to rise in the next few decades. However, when we look at the science behind the production of sugar, and then compare it with our biological oven, that is our body, which also makes its own sugar. The only difference is the name we give to it and the formula that puts it into effect. In this chapter, I will take you through the various steps of making different types of sugar, as well as study what sugar does to our body. Hopefully, it will make it easier for you to understand the complex science, which brings glucose into being in the first place.

3.1. HOW IS SUGAR MADE?

First of all, let us look at how we extract sugar from sugarcane and beet sugar. It is the most widely known form of sucrose that we see in our kitchen cupboards that comes: white, brown or golden. These are the sugar crystals that you add to your tea and/or coffee, cereals, cake recipes, etc. It looks like a simple bag of sugar, does it not? However, there is a complex process to produce the white sugar that we are so familiar with. First of all, there is the harvesting, extraction, separation, and evaporation followed by crystallization, centrifugation, and purification.
The Sugar Association includes this simplified version of how to make sugar on their webpage:

"All sugar is made by first extracting sugar juice from sugar beet or sugar cane plants., and from there, many types of sugar can be produced. Through slight adjustments in the process of cleaning, crystallizing and drying the sugar and varying the level of molasses, different sugar varieties are possible. Sugars of various crystal sizes provide unique functional characteristics that make the sugar suitable for different foods and beverages. Sugar color is primarily determined by the amount of molasses remaining on or added to the crystals, giving pleasurable flavors and altering moisture. Heating sugar also changes the color and flavor (yum, caramel!). Some types of sugar are used only by the food industry and are not available in the supermarket."

Not only have they made the whole process of extracting sugar juice, while turning it into sugar cane seem simple, but they purposely use inviting and positive language intended to draw you into consuming it. Therefore, I am going to take this process and explain it differently. I will not be biased, but I will explain it in better detail, so you can really see how to make sugar. First of all, the sucrose that we digest is something that derives in plants, which they produce in the process of photosynthesis in the leaves; it then collects and stores in the plant's stalk. Sugar cane has one of the highest forms of concentrated sugar where the stems can grow up to 20 ft. tall. However, sugar cane is very damaging to the earth's soil because it needs a lot of minerals to grow. It also requires a specific climate to grow properly, which is a tropical one – lots of rain and hot weather. Over time, sugarcane can completely drain the ground of all its minerals, leaving it dry and infertile. Sugar cane is renewable; it does not need replanting every time a new crop wants to be made. You simply cut the stalks at the base, leaving room for the grass to grow out again and produce a fresh harvest from the old crop.

In the process of photosynthesis, roots work to pull water and minerals up from the ground, while the leaves take in carbon dioxide. The plant's leaves' cells, called chlorophyll, also absorb sunlight. You might remember this process when you studied at school as a plant's natural lifecycle. However, did you know that it is also set to produce the plant's natural sugar? It is a natural sugary juice collected in the inside of the stem, as hydrated carbon. It is also known as a pure and sweetened form of carbohydrate. In other words:

UV SUNLIGHT ENERGY + CARBON DIOXIDE + WATER = SUCROSE

Or in its scientific formula:

C12H22O11
(12 atoms of carbon to 22 atoms of hydrogen and 11 atoms of oxygen)

However, you can also break sugar down into these two components:

FRUCTOSE + GLUCOSE = SUCROSE

Fructose is the natural sugar present in fruit and some root vegetables, and glucose is the sugar we produce in our bloodstream. Therefore, sucrose is a double concentration of sugar, which links these two components. Funnily enough, both fructose and glucose appear as the same formula, which is:

***$C_6H_{12}O_6$. ***

Sugar comes in lots of different forms, which includes the sugar that we produce in our bloodstream. Our body is biologically designed to regulate its own sugar levels. It is in our DNA, just like it is in plant's DNA, to produce sugar. It could be why we are so attracted to the taste because it is very addictive too. However, this addictive quality, which sugar has, is even more dangerous. When we produce sugar as glucose in a process called Glycogenolysis, which I will elaborate on more lately. For now, let us stay on the subject where we extract the sucrose out of plants, specifically looking at sugarcane and sugar beet.

The harvest of sugarcane is cut using a sugarcane harvester, which was appropriately developed in the 1930s by Mr. Wurtele, inventing this innovatory machinery to cut the sugarcane to the base stalk more efficiently. However, it also strips the stalk leaves and shreds up the solid, hard stem into smaller pieces where it is stored in a container, which is then taken back to the mill - that were once, and in some cases still, powered by big wind-turbines. There the extraneous process of extracting the sucrose juice from the sugar cane begins where we turn the sweetened milk into the small, dry crystals of sugar we know and love today.

I am going to explain to you this neat extraction-production process in 15 essential stages. Therefore, when the truckloads of beaten sugar cane stalks are shipped in their kilos to the giant production mill - it endures a linear process before it reaches the shelves of our supermarket, or condiment cupboard:

    1)   Firstly they wash the sugar cane stalks down

    2)   Then they cut them into shreds

    3)   The stalks are crushed and pressed with big metal rollers to squeeze out the juice, which then drains into the separator

    4)   In the separator, it removes the fibers and impurities

5)   Then the purified liquid collects into an enormous evaporator pot, which is heated over a burning fiery furnace that uses the separated waste fibers of the sugar that was separated in stage four - as fuel for the evaporating process

6)   With the heat of the vapor - caramelization takes place, producing a golden syrup, which thickens over the boiling water.

7)   The syrup is left to cool and dry

8)   A crystallization process is started by adding crystals to the cool liquid syrup.

9)   The moist crystalized sugar is transferred to a centrifuge where a process of centrifugation takes place by spinning the sugar fast in circular dial pots with centrifugal force that squeeze all the remaining liquid out

10)   Sugar crystals are left to dry some more

11)   Further purification of the sugar takes place

12)   De-colorization of the sugar produces white cane sugar, which is the most popular form of sugar.

13)   Re-crystallization - one more time after it has dried!

14)   Dried again in a granulator.

15)   Sugar is packaged and branded for exportation.

Sugar comes in crystallized form in three different types, which depends on the stage of refinement towards the end of production. Turbinado or cane sugar is partially refined sugar. Brown sugar contains some of the caramel molasses coating still, which is produced in the caramelization stage and gives it a distinct taste and brown color. Finally, white sugar is what goes through all fifteen stages of production and passes the final granulating stage. This complex extraction is not only necessary to extract the sweetened juice. It also works to heighten the sugar concentration in the evaporation stage, which makes it even more lethal if we consume it in large quantities. However, this is just one of the sugars we know of because there are plenty of other forms of sugar. However, most of them, if not all, should be consumed in short supply, even fruit that has sugar in its fructose form, and I will explain to you why.

Again, although we don't need sugar, it has become an essential commodity to food production, as well as cooking. Sugar is especially good at enhancing flavor, as well as aroma and texture. When used in cooking, its caramelization properties are suitable for browning or glazing meat, and other foods. Finally, it will also retain moisture and preserve the freshness of food.

3.2. TYPES OF SUGAR

Sugar comes in its purest form, which is **$C_6H_{12}O_6$ ** in three different types: fructose, galactose and glucose. Galactose and glucose are the sugar, which we in our bloodstream, as well as other members of the animal family. Fructose is in most plant-based products, such as fruit and vegetables, which give them their rich, sweet taste that essentially makes them excellent sources of natural energy. It is the fructose in corn, which they use to make high fructose corn syrup that they use to flavor most processed foods. Interestingly, vegetables tend to have a higher level of fructose. Sugar cane and sugar beet are the most highly concentrated vegetables, followed by beetroot, carrot and sweet potato. Apricots, peaches, and pineapple provide the highest concentrations of fructose levels in fruits. Fructose is one of the healthiest forms of eating sugar because it does not increase your blood sugar level dangerously high. It works naturally with the glucose in your body to produce natural, healthy levels of energy. However, if consumed in large amounts, then it can produce excess body fat and also trigger a dependency on sugary products found in other products. That is particularly dangerous if you are already addicted or dependent on sugar.

Sugar comes in more concentrated forms, such as lactose, which is again a natural form of sugar produced in mammal's milk. Sugar also comes in the form of honey, which is a liquid form of sugar that bees naturally make. They take the sugary secretions from plant leaves and turn them into honeydew through a process of natural excretion and regurgitation. There are various syrups, such as maple and treacle syrup, as well as high fructose corn syrup, also known as HFCS. HFCS is a sweetener made from corn starch that is broken down into glucose and supplements fructose by converting some of the glucose down by glucose isomerase. It is a factory processed form of creating sucrose, which is much more cost-effective but also more lethal to our bodies. Although the sugar federation has stated that it is tested and completely harmless to our bodies, this is more than skeptical and over the years has been proved adversely inaccurate.

A further stage in the sugar process is the fermenting stage, which produces alcohol. Ethanol fermentation is the process of converting sugars, such as glucose, fructose, and sucrose into a compound cellular energy, which produces ethanol and carbon dioxide. The absence of oxygen means that yeasts are created, which are efficient in the process of breaking down enzymes, typical in the process of fermentation. It is also a process they use to help raise the yeast in the bread-making process. Alcohol is not only high in sugar and very addictive, but it is also very harmful and creates adverse effects on your mental and physical state. When we metabolize grains and sucrose in its pure form, we absorb 80% into our body cells and our liver absorbs the remaining 20%. However, the metabolism of alcohol is in reverse, meaning that the liver absorbs 80 % of the glucose. Therefore, when we consume alcohol in excess over a long time, it almost always leads to liver disease.

Alcohol also induces your kidneys to eliminate liquid towards the bladder as if we have excess water, which causes dehydration. The liver does not get the water it needs to process the toxins in the alcohol. Alternatively, it takes excess liquid from the brain, which is why we begin to feel light-headed. As you drink more and more, this feeling will worsen. It then has adverse effects on mood swings and temperament. The next day you may also suffer from headaches and a sense of dehydration, amongst other side effects like nausea and tiredness. It is your body repairing itself and your liver working hard to hydrate your body back to its natural biological state. It is one thing that we forget!

Our body is a biological oven of complex natural processes set there for a reason. It has evolved over millennia eating a particular diet in a certain way. However, this diet is the reverse to how the majority of us feed ourselves today. We forget that we are what we eat and everything we consume, we must digest to excrete then. Food, or nutrition from food, is what we need to keep the natural process of our body working; it feeds us with energy to carry out our overall body s daily routine. There are certain nutrients our body needs more than others, namely vitamins, proteins, omega three, and fatty acids that you find in saturated fats. Excess sugar and carbohydrates are toxic to our body, especially in high supply, yet it makes up a more significant part of our diet at present. That is especially after the recommendations we were given in the late 20th century. In other words, for the last 20 years, most of us have been poisoning our bodies.

3.3. SUGAR IN OUR BODY - GLUCOSE

So why is sugar toxic? You might have had the impression that we needed sugar. Sugar is in our blood, is it not? Well, yes, it is. However, that is because, like plants, we produce our own sugar. Everything we eat, as soon as it passes our mouth is no longer meat, or fish, vegetables, cake, or your favorite comfort food anymore. We might have a separate taste for each food type, and when it makes contact with our palette, it sends a message to our brain telling us what we have eaten, but also whether we like it or not. However, as soon as it passes down our throat, it becomes one collective thing, which is glucose, and the key source of energy in our body. Therefore, when our brain tells us whether or not we like something, it often deceives us. It might not necessarily mean if we like it, the food is good for us. Then again, we might eat something we find repulsive like a Brussels sprout, for example. Do you remember when your grandparents would serve you up a ration of Brussels sprouts on your plate, and you would turn your nose up at them? It would feel like torture eating them because they taste so bitter. However, they are full of minerals and nutrients, and they are probably one of the most healthy things you can feed your body.

On the other hand, sugar is not. When we eat sucrose *sugar,* then we are overfeeding ourselves sugar. Our bloodstream exceeds its normal sugar levels, which is when sugar is intoxicating. The liver and pancreas are vital in regulating our blood sugar levels, which involve the release of insulin.

When our body requires more energy, or more glucose in the blood, then it will ask for more food. When your body starts to produce too much glucose, then it begins to store it as glycerol in your liver, in a process called glycogenolysis. It does this with the help of insulin, which is a hormone that you release when your body sees that there is excess glucose in the bloodstream. It is secreted in the pancreas and helps lower your blood sugar levels, so that this glucose can be absorbed and stored in your body cells and muscle mass. That way, when you need more fuel to burn for energy, you have it on the ready! For example, when you sleep, you need that extra fuel to keep your body clock ticking by. You are unconscious dreaming the night away, while your body is working twenty-four seven.

Now when you eat sugar or carbohydrates in excess, and the glycerol you have stored for energy fuel does not get burnt off, then it gets stored as body fat instead. It is not saturated fats that produce excess body fat; it is carbohydrates and sugar. They provide calories and no nutrients. The excess consumption of these two ingredients, which is typical in most cultures and dietary menus today, but which we also see advertised everywhere - on billboards, supermarkets, or the television: pizza, pasta, sandwiches, burgers, soft drinks, juice, baked beans, etc. The list is endless! However, all these products do is supplement our blood with excess glucose (sugar), which our body does not need. It completely interrupts our body cycle, which has had a specific mechanism of working evolving over millennia eating the same way.

When the amount of sugar that you consume is more considerable than what your body cells, muscle mass and liver can store, then the liver will turn it into body fat. Body fat is made up of triglycerides, which are three fatty acid molecules to one molecule of glycerol. So, without the one unit of glycerol, which you produce when you have excess sugar in your system, then your body would not store fat. The trouble with body fat is that you can carry on accumulating at a tremendous rate. You can store fat on top fat without stopping. That is why you see people reach such immense sizes. Records show that the heaviest man weighs over half a ton, or the equivalent of 600kg at twenty-two years of age. As you can imagine, his health factors are in a life-threatening condition, and he has been hospitalized for treatment needing urgent help to lose weight.

It is straightforward, though, because all he must do is eliminate carbohydrates and sugar from his diet, and then he will naturally lose weight in the right way. Too many people are given the wrong guidelines to lose weight because doctors and scientists are still protecting their reputation for providing the false information, which they recommended to everyone to cut saturated fats out of our diet and supplement it with carbohydrates. In turn, this recommendation has made over 50% of the US population obese, as well as insulin resistant. In other words, the body produces too much insulin, which raises our blood sugar levels out of control those risks harming our hearts. It is what most of us recognize to be Diabetes type 2.

Why is it then, which people are recommended to eat low-fat diets, rather than cut out the sugar? When you look at the low-fat, supposedly healthy, processed meal options, there is little fat, yet it is still high in sugar dosage. In light of what I have just shared with you, can you see these people losing weight? Maybe, that is why, even though there are more diets around than ever before, obesity is still dangerously on the rise. Nothing has been done about limiting the amount of sugar added to dietary products. Instead, in the same decade that *The Times* released its article, insisting people cut saturated fats out of their diet. Then sugar in the form of High Fructose Corn Syrup (used by big food brands in almost everything) was permitted by the Foods Chemicals Codex to be used as an ingredient with no dosage limitations. In other words, companies were allowed to add as much sugar as they liked, which they did!

Why? Because it is addictive.

Therefore, the more people eat it, the more they want it.

3.4. ADDICTION TO SUGAR

"Sugar is something nobody needs, but everyone craves."

Have you ever had a craving for a sweet delight? Do you need that extra teaspoon of sugar in your tea or coffee to tickle your taste buds? You may find that once you start eating sugary snacks, you find you just can't stop! Do you think you might have an addiction to sugar? Most of you may believe you do not, but sometimes it could only be a glass of sugary soft drink, or a slice of bread you wish to nibble on. Do you think it is your body telling you that you are hungry, or that it wants sugar? The answer to this question is simple.

What is it that you are craving? Could it be possible that the craving you are experiencing seeks out sugar? It will not be because your body needs it, but because your mind desires the satisfaction, it gets when you taste it.

When we eat sugar or any food, which we sweeten with sugar, it instantly sends a message to our brain that we like it. The message is sent to the reward part of our brain, which sends off neurons of positive reinforcement, called endorphins. This reward sensitization is what we read as a craving that we want more of it. However, remember how the mind deceives us; it is not our body that needs it to survive, but your mind deceiving you. However, with time the craving may become a habit, which upon repeated exposure with the pattern effect becomes what we call: an addiction. We seek out the experience of reward that we get by indulging in it till it becomes a compulsive behavior that we expose ourselves to it as much as we can to tide over what are called the withdrawal symptoms. Effectively, over time through frequent exposure, our body becomes dependent on the sensation that it gives us. It could be dependent on a substance like sugar, or alcohol (which is merely fermented sugar), or it could also be a behavior even. Addictions to sex and gambling are the most popular forms of compulsive behavioral disorders. Whereas sugar is one of the most unnoticed, deadly, and devours the most numerous cases of addicts, which is nearly all of us.

I would not be surprised if sugar were one of mans' first addictions; it *"is something nobody needs but everyone craves."* We never needed to taste sugar, but we did. We produced it on a monumental scale, all because, when countries first started discovering it, they were instantly intrigued by its taste. It provided a feeling of reward in people that meant people craved more. This addictive quality encouraged people to travel over borders and discover new lands so that they could cultivate products, such as sugar, tobacco, and coffee, all of which require hot, tropical climates. The Americas were discovered, The New World Order was put into place, and people were allowed to indulge in their desires (addictions), as much as they liked. However, this controlled compulsive behavior has adverse effects on our health.

First of all, it is very controlling, and over time the effects where the neurons need to balance out again when the sensation of reward wears off, effectively leaves us feeling worse. When you imbalance your endorphins in such a way, then to regulate them back to normal, you start getting a reverse feeling of 'doom and gloom.' Over time, your mood becomes more unstable when you are not indulging in that 'guilty pleasure.' Therefore, you indulge in it more frequently until it becomes dangerously harmful to your physical health, especially in the case of sugar. As you saw before, an excess of sugar consumption is what causes our body to turn fatty acids from carbohydrates, amongst other things, into body fat, which you store at an unlimited rate if you do not burn that fat off. The process then releases more insulin to calm down the blood sugar levels, and with time this can affect your sugar levels so that they are harder to regulate. It will eventually develop into Diabetes type 2, and then heart disease, which is known to be extremely deadly.

What is worse is that when you eat any type of fructose, it also shuts down the part of your brain that tells you that you are full. That makes the sucrose even more destructive because you will carry on eating sugary snacks without your mind registering that you have eaten at all. How many times have we indulged in cake, or a fast food meal, and we feel like we have eaten a lot? However, half an hour later, we are hungry again. It is not because we have not eaten enough; it is because our brain craves more. That is why when we drink sugary drinks with a meal; it does not fill us up like we think it should. Instead, it will inspire us to eat more, mainly if what we are eating includes sugar in it. Sugar asks for more sugar, which could be why we were attracted to it in the first place.

However, an addiction to sugar is not so much a guilty pleasure but a deadly treasure. It is one that was discovered on a small island of paradise in the South Pacific, some three thousand years ago. It brought money and fame to countries worldwide. However, it also brought shame and misfortune. Most of us are also unaware of just how toxic sugar is.

Another thing we are unaware of is just how much sugar we eat on a day to day basis or the grand infrastructure of business we keep alive depending on our addiction to sugar. It is the very reason why they were allowed to publicize statements reprimanding saturated fats from our diet in the 1970s and 80s. It is also why the Sugar Association went unnoticed funding one of the destructive false publications in 1967, via the voice of three untrustworthy Harvard science students. It is also why Ancel Keys was allowed to rise to stardom with his highly inaccurate study that changed the face of dietary nutrition advice, forever! It became wrong advice for what then would happen to the sugar business? We will look at this in our next chapter, but first let us have a quick look at what is our recommended daily intake of sugar.

3.4. DAILY RECOMMENDED SUGAR DOSE

Now we have looked at what sugar does to our body, and we have seen that an excess of sugar is deadly. We are going to look in more detail at just how harmful later on. It will be something that develops with time. As you expose yourself to more sugar, then you are not only going to crave it more, but you are going to digest it differently. Your biological oven of a body starts to work a little slower as you get older, which is when you see most people begin to put more weight on, say from their mid-thirties onwards.

It is always good to limit your consumption of sugar or products with sugar in it. They might also include any chemical derivatives of sugar like High Fructose Corn Syrup, which is a popular ingredient used in processed foods, but also added in excessive amounts. We are going to look at this later. However, let us look first at the daily intake of sugar by the average person. In America, the average person consumes 25-30 teaspoons of sugar a day. It

is the equivalent of 40-50 kilos of sugar a year. Fortunately, due to the increased health risks correlated to consuming too much sugar, The *World Health Organization* advises that we should eat no more than twelve teaspoons of sugar a day. However, the *American Heart Association* recommends we should east just six teaspoons of sugar a day.
Now when I say teaspoons of sugar, I don t mean teaspoons of sugar literally like what you put in coffee. However, one or two of these we should also include in our daily limit. What I mean is, the equivalent of eight teaspoons, which might be in yogurt, bread, chocolate, cake, tomato ketchup, etc. One thing I am going to reveal to you in this next chapter is just how excessive our sugar menu is with products that have an exceeding amount of sugar that we didn't even know had it in them. A tin of baked beans, for example, how many teaspoons do you think?
 Well, you're going to be shocked because if you eat a tin of baked beans, then you have very nearly reached your daily limit. It rests at six teaspoons of sugar. For those of you shocked at this fact and wondering how it is even possible when baked beans are supposed to be savory, sometimes *healthy* snack options. Well, they are not! There is, in fact, a secret formula - a balancing ingredient, which can tone down the overly sweet taste of sugar but still keep consumption of sugar as high as possible. Fortunately, with the aid of the Food Codex in1981, food companies were allowed to add as much sugar as possible, regardless of the health warnings. They were fast and efficiently tucked under the carpet using the powerful tool of the media, as well as the authoritative image that the doctors, scientists, and governing bodies embodied. In effect, they sponsored the multi-million dollar business, which is now sugar to reach its level of high profitability. They did this by keeping a thick blindfold wrapped tightly around our eyes. It is what I compared to you before with The Matrix, and also Alice and Wonderland's trip down the rabbit hole. Now, do you want to see why?...

3.5. THERE ARE TIMES TO EAT SUGAR

In this next chapter, I am going to discuss the importance of picking the right time to eat sugar. I want to bring you back to the idea that your body works on specific patterns, as well as times. For example, when our body turns glucose into glycerol, then it secretes insulin, which will lower your blood sugar levels. Insulin stays working in your system for two to three hours at a time before it starts to regulate the blood levels back to normal. Therefore, it is advisable to leave a few hours between snacking and meal times. It is also essential to consume less sugary products in one go because our liver, which is our glucose-making machine, finds it harder to metabolize fructose, over other food types like fats, vitamins, and carbohydrates. There is also a risk that if you eat products that have a high level of fructose or sucrose, you will put weight on. They have a high concentration of triglycerides, which can form into body fat when your liver cannot find anywhere else to store it. Therefore, if you frequently snack out on 'sweets,' you will become obese, possibly risk suffering from diabetes type-2, as well as damage your liver and cause other health-related issues. Diabetes type-2 has been directly linked to the abnormal sugar levels in your blood caused by your body, producing too much insulin.

Not only is it vital that you limit your sugar in dietary products, as well as the frequency that you eat it. You should also avoid eating sugar in the morning and late at night. In the morning, your body wakes after a long night of working hard at metabolizing the food you gave it the day before. It will already be high in glucose. A breakfast, which is enriched with saturated fats, will supplement the glucose and kick start your liver and pancreas, turning it into glycerol. Unfortunately, because most of us are unaware that we are addicted to sugar, then most of us will crave something sugary. A bowl of sweetened cereal with sweetened coffee, or a custard cream donut even. However, putting toxins in your system so early in the day, especially sugar, will have adverse effects on your natural metabolizing process. Alternatively, if you snack on 'sweets' at night, then you can interrupt your body clock. Sugary snacks and food causes an adrenalin rush that often leaves you feeling excited, and sometimes nervous. These side-effects are seen at their worst when you go to sleep. People you consume high amounts of sugar, especially at night, are more likely to have interrupted sleep, or suffer from sleep apnea. It can then have further adverse effects on your health, causing anxiety and depression, amongst other issues.

There are some forms of sugar, or fructose, which are healthier for you. The fructose in fruit and vegetables is much better for you because the concentration of sugar is lower than in other dietary products. However, again you have to be careful how much you eat and when you eat it. Yes, even fruit. Unless you are going to burn the energy off when you eat the fruit, then over eating it could also turn it into body fat, when you cannot use it.

Finally, before I move onto my next subject of debate surrounding our favorite condiment to self-destruction, I want to look at when it is the correct time to give children sugar. Well, if you were going to eliminate any risk factors caused by excess sugar intake, then I would not give children sugar at all. I guess if they did not get a taste for it, then they would never feel the desire to eat more. However, that would be an ideology that is impossible and slightly cruel. We are all allowed a guilty 'sweet' pleasure once in a while. However, remember, children are susceptible to getting addicted to sugar very quickly.

Furthermore, the effects of sugar are also more harmful. Their bodies are much smaller than ours, and they are still developing. Therefore, if you feed children high-levels of sugar, then you are effectively poisoning them. This fact has been made evident with the controversially high numbers of Diabetes type-2, as well as obesity in children, even younger than ten years old. Furthermore, the adrenalin rush that we adults get when we consume sugar may feel energetic. However, it takes more effect after a child consumes sugar. It is an instant reaction to the sugar rush that in some children, if not most, will cause adverse behavior, including mood swings and symptoms similar to Attention Deficit Hyperactivity Disorder (ADHD). ADHD is a mental health disorder that can cause above-normal levels of hyperactive and impulsive behavior. In recent decades the diagnosis for this disease in children has gone up, which has then resulted in doctors advising parents to medicate their children (as young as 3/4 years old) with drugs to regulate their behavior and energy levels. Unfortunately, many doctors are too quick to diagnose child patients with ADHD in the United States without actually studying the child's diet, or the effect that high levels of sugar might also be doing to their diet. It might be a simple case of cutting out the sugar, where you save yourself a lifetime of medical bills. However, you will also benefit your child's future mental health that is likely to have adverse effects from taking strong medication at such a young age, especially if he did not need to.

Therefore, not only is it essential to limit your sugar intake to six teaspoons of sugar a day. I would also be careful when you decide to eat, but also maybe lowering the count of sugar dosage you give your little ones. You are responsible for their health, and providing a proper, nutritional diet that should not include any sugar, let alone be full with it.

4

Excess Sugar

Well, we know now that once people with money and power caught sight of the tasty sweetener that appeared as a *"reed which gives honey without bees."* It was as far back as 510 BC by the King of Persia who stepped foot on India's soil, and saw its money-making potential. With the move of sugar to the Americas, then we saw a multi-billion business put into place around the age of industrialization. Not only did sugar become amenable to everyone, which allowed for even more marketing and a higher volume of sales. It was supplied with inventions that eased the production of sugar. With modernization, big corporate food industries took the opportunity to exploit sugar to a great extent, especially when they realized just how addictive sugar is. However, skeptical the health issues were that had started arising at the beginning of the 20th century, they were soon shunned with the advice given by Ancel Keys, and consequently, many doctors and nurses. The notice that appeared in the 1984 edition of *The Times* magazine, which had been reiterated in numerous other magazines in the decades leading up that: "Cholesterol is deadly," insisted that we should not eat saturated fats.

Furthermore, the rise of the artificial sweetener, which became most fashionably known as high fructose corn syrup, also took the eye away from the public. People did not associate the name on the food label with sugar. Therefore, they could add this ingredient to their hearts' desire. In the meantime, more food brands started to appear on the scene who took the opportunity to use sugar as their main ingredient. It was highly profitable because it was so addictive. Companies encouraged the addictive properties to keep their sales soaring high, regardless of the health issues. What mattered was that the greater parts of their consumers were unaware of it. Therefore, in the early 70s, when a man called Dr. Howard Moskowitz came up with *The Bliss Point* Theory. It allowed for the food industry to take full advantage of being able to add as much sugar as they liked because they could balance it out with salt. The more sugar they added to a recipe, then the more palpable it tasted. What we didn't realize is that again, the sugar blinded us. However, this time it is not the wrong nutritional advice that they are giving us, but the amount of sugar we are actually ingesting into our system.

I am going to reveal to you just how much! Then I will also tell you why the food industries are doing this. They do it to protect the system. This system is what Morpheus explains to Neo, as a somewhat controlling hierarchy that became possible with the rising power of the voice of the media. However, there are more parties involved that control from the top, and it's all there to fuel one thing, which is money and business.

4.1. THE BLISS POINT THEORY

The Bliss Point theory was an innovative invention for the food industry, made by Dr. Howard Moskowitz. It quite literally means finding the 'level of happiness' in food so that when we taste it, we get that rush of sheer delight. As Dr. Moskowitz stated with his discovery that he found: "the level where you like that product the most." He desired to find the formulaic ingredient that optimized the palpability of food. He saw sugar to have incredibly effective responses, along with salt. It is interesting to know that Dr. Moskowitz graduated from Harvard University. However, not as a scientist, bio-chemist, or nutritionist, he graduated with a diploma in market research and psychology. Moskowitz might have studied the reward system of the brain as a way of providing the ideal marketing tool. When he realized that people were susceptible to being addicted to sugar, he probably saw an excellent opportunity to exploit this *magic* ingredient, which was aided with the invention of high fructose corn syrup, as well as the media articles, which laid the blame on fat. You might be starting to see a significant connection. Although we have been made blind to it, there has been a whole interconnection of different discoveries and devices, which paved the way for even more success allowing sugar to make millions of dollars while it harmed millions of lives.

However, the 'level of happiness' in the Bliss Point theory is not met by adding only sugar. As you can imagine, when you taste a cup of coffee or tea that you added too much sugar to, it would appear too sweet. However, Dr. Moskowitz theorizes with the Bliss Point that if you then add salt, then it will balance out the sweet taste with some added bitterness, and hey presto! You have a wonderfully sugary, but still unnoticed addictive product on the shelves for millions of people to purchase and consume by the metric ton. It became implemented as the primary ingredient in most processed drinks and foods. Companies that specialize in making products, swearing by the *bliss point* formula, will have conference meetings to decide the ideal 'level of sweetness' prescribed by Dr. Moskowitz. For example, a group of company directors and specialists are presented with three different versions of the same recipe. However, each one will contain varying levels of concentrated sugar; say three, four, or five teaspoons. They will then vote, which tastes the best, or has reached the ideal *bliss point*. It is the chosen recipe they will use for that particular product line. It is a vital procedure companies like Coca Cola and Cadburys implement, which allows their sales to shoot out the roof. Then with market branding and logos that have become iconic in today's society. There is no doubt in thinking that Dr. Moskowitz was the pioneer for market research, as well as product branding. And how do you reach people's attention most effectively?... Through the control of their psyche, and what better way to control them than by their reward system.

4.2. THE RISE OF THE ARTIFICIAL SWEETENER

Now even though spokespeople and scientists like Ancel Keys were working hard at identifying saturated fats being bad for your heart, medical professionals were also keen to recommend people to eat less sugar. However, because cases of diabetes rose in the 1960s, along with other health issues connected to an excessive intake of sugar, then it drove companies who were attached to the Sugar Association to experiment in the market of artificial sweeteners. It was a much more cost-effective way of producing highly concentrated sweetened syrup in high volume where the factories could control the levels of sweetness to their desire. However, to start with, the Food Codex Federation was quick at identifying the health risks to the first artificial sweeteners that appeared on the scene.

Firstly, Calcium cyclamate appeared in the first soda drinks in 1952, but it was soon banned for being carcinogenic. Then in 1965, another sweetener appeared and also disappeared, just as fast called Aspartame (NutraSweet). Finally, in 1967, they discovered high fructose corn syrup, also known as corn syrup or HFCS. It derives from corn starch, which is a highly concentrated grain food type. Fortunately, corn was in abundant supply in the United States, and it can grow anywhere, but also tall. The first producers of the artificial sweetener appeared in the 1970s, namely the Clinton Corn Processing Company and the Japanese Agency of Industrial Science and Technology. High fructose corn syrup (HFCS) was highly profitable, especially when they began to tax sugar high in 1977; they had to save their costs somewhere. HFCS was able to stay in production because of the great testament, which was made by the Sugar Association that it did not promote any health risks to people. However, this has proven to be a false claim again to protect their 'secret' formula.

As we have learned, high fructose corn syrup (HFCS) is a highly concentrated glucose-fructose formula made from corn starch. In the process of production, the starch, which already contains fructose, is then broken down partly into glucose as until it reaches a relative ratio of 42% fructose and 53% glucose. This process is done by mixing hydrochloric acid with industrial made enzymes that are produced using bacteria, for example -amylase produced from Bacillus app. The enzyme hydrolyzes corn starch to smaller chain dextrin and oligosaccharides. A second enzyme, glucoamylase, produced from Aspergillus (fungi) breaks down the dextrin and oligosaccharides, leaving the artificial sugar glucose. It all sounds rather complicated, or scientific, does it not? Well, that is because it is. Where the 19th century saw improvements in productions with new machines that inventors came up with, then the late 20th century saw science take the floor. Scientific research, which was paid for by the government and industries, such as the Sugar Association, created new formulas that could be compared to natural flavors. The only thing is they were more adaptable, but also unnatural still. Our digestive system has never been exposed to them before. Therefore, how were we to know if it was good for us or not?

It is only in recent years that more investigation has been carried out because the cases in diabetes and obesity have risen to reach shocking numbers in the last forty years since it was implemented to the human diet. It was not just tested out on a few things either; it was added to nearly everything. They went hand in hand with the discovery of HFCS, so did hundreds of new manufacturing companies specializing in processed, ready-made meals start appearing. To this day, it stands that 99% of companies that specialize in the mass-production of processed foods use high fructose corn syrup as their main 'secret' ingredient. However, it is often written in different forms again to distract you from seeing it in the ingredients. For example, you might find it written as: HFCS-90, HFCS-42, and also HFCS-55.

The production of high fructose corn syrup was aided with the discovery of the Bliss Point theory discovered by Dr. Howard Moskowitz in the early 70s. It involved finding the taste with the best 'level of happiness' by adding lots of sugar, which they could balance out with salt. Although it was considered a person's level of satisfaction, it then became their health risk, and the food industry's *bliss point*. Notably, in 1981 when the Food Codex Federation allowed for people to add unlimited amounts of sweetened additives to processed foods. It meant companies could now add all the sugar they liked; the more, the better! Only because it got people addicted to sugar quicker, and the product itself, which means people would buy it in the bulk load - and that they did. However, they also put on pounds of fat by the bulk load too!

In recent years health advisors have documented extreme risks to our health from ingesting too many products with high levels of high fructose corn syrup. These include heart disease, high blood pressure, obesity, diabetes, liver failure, Alzheimer's disease, etc. Here are the reasons why:

    1) It adds an abnormal amount of fructose to your diet, which your liver finds hard to break down into glucose

    2) It increases the chance of fatty liver disease from producing too much fat, which happens when the glucose levels are too high. They cannot be stored elsewhere in muscle mass, or body cells.

    3) It increases your risk of putting on weight or becoming obese because fructose is known to promote the accumulation of visceral fat, which is harmful to your organs

    4) Excessive intake of HFCS is also linked to diabetes type 2 where you become insulin resistant where your body can no longer metabolize food properly

5) Overconsumption of fructose present in HFCS drives inflammation, which is known to increase the risk of other serious diseases developing like gout, heart disease, etc.

Unfortunately, once again, we were conned into thinking that high fructose corn syrup was good for us in the late 20th century. It allowed for another fatal mistake to be made in the whole scheme of food production. However, we are the only victims at the end of the day because the food companies, which implement this ingredient, make millions from it. We follow suit and buy it unknown to what it is doing to us, which is killing us. We are fooled by the Bliss Point companies who are able to disguise how much HFCS is in products, like soda drinks - the equivalent of 10 teaspoons of sugar to one single serving. However, we are also blinded by the fact that we are being bombarded with temptation and advertisements every day to buy and ingest this harmful artificial ingredient. How do we stay away from the health issues caused by this ingredient? Well, it is easy. Firstly, try and avoid buying processed foods and drinks. Go back to cooking everything from scratch, even your pasta sauce, which also has high concentrations of HFCS

We are in a modern toxic world where we have to question everything we read, see and hear, even when it is presented to us officially. There is always a chance there is a deep, dark secret behind it covering something up to product a massive money-making industry. Well, you sort of hope that this is not the case. It would be sad if we could not trust anyone, although there is no harm in being weary.

4.3. HOW MANY TEASPOONS OF SUGAR?

Now that Dr. Moskowitz had discovered the Bliss Point theory, then by 1981, the Food Codex also allowed for companies to add as much sugar as they saw 'fit.' People are afraid that sugar and fat might harm them. Sugar appears in lots of different forms, such as high fructose corn syrup. As you can imagine, food companies took the opportunity to add as much sugar to products as possible. It meant that they would become addicted to them, but also crave more, so buy more. As we looked at before, sugar was the ideal marketing tool. Therefore, it was added in copious amounts. However, most of us do not realize just how much. So now, I want to take you through a simple look at some of our favorite high-street dietary products that we put in our shopping trolleys - and see just how much sugar is in them. Let us go back and use our teaspoon metric measurements.

Remember that the American Heart Association recommended that we only have six teaspoons of sugar a day. Then when you start to see just how much sugar is in everything, you can begin to realize how we reach to exceed twenty teaspoons of sugar a day. You can also begin to see why there is such an epidemic of Diabetes type 2 and obesity in many countries. Now what you are about to discover may be shocking to some of you. However, when you are made aware of it, only then can you begin to make a change today. You can start limiting the sugar in your diet by limiting the amount of products, like these in your diet. Now I will take you through a re-run of some of your favorite products and look at just how much sugar is in them:

SHOPPING LIST

Can of Coca Cola 50ml   …….. 10 (teaspoons of sugar)

Glass of apple juice 7
Glass of milk 3
Pint of Beer. 9
Flavored water. 5
Heinz Baked Beans (tin) 10
Heinz Tomato Ketchup. (1 tablespoon) 1
Loaf of white bread. 10
Average bowl of fiber cereal 6
Pizza 8
'Healthy-living' low-fat ready-made meal. 6

It is a small selection of your favorite processed food products that you might find yourself eating every day without much regard to how much sugar is in them. Do you see that most of these products also exceed your daily intake of sugar? There is no need for it. Well, think about where you might be in the next twenty to thirty years, maybe even less if you have followed this diet already for a while? There is only so much your liver will take, or your heart will take. Remember that what you eat becomes a part of you, and it will take effect, whether positively or adversely it depends on you. You decide what you eat and what you feed your body. We shy away from the future because it seems so far away, but every day that passes is another day that you poison your body if you decide to cave into your craving for sugar. It isn't easy either when you have these all-time amazing and addictive sweetened products at your fingertips, often cheaper than if you buy natural food these days. I wonder why?

What is worse, you have the names branded everywhere: when you walk down the shopping aisles, open your kitchen cupboard or anyone's for that matter. Then you go to a bar or a restaurant- you see them! You see them on the big, billboards outside your office windows and on the way home from work. You see them on posters in the shop windows, in the metro stations, on the buses. Then when you get back home to relax finally and watch some television, say your favorite series; it gets interrupted every five minutes with video advertisements about them. It is also the time you're your most susceptible to caving into your cravings. Branding is everywhere, and companies involved in the sugar industry, especially the retail food production companies, pay heavily in advertising to keep themselves seen and heard by everyone, so everyone consumes them. It is the final key to the link - propaganda markets and advertises addictive products. Therefore, they can control us under their system. It is a little like *the Matrix* that we live in!

Is it not?

4.4. BRANDING SUGAR

So I am trying to advise you here to give up sugar in your diet because it is incredibly unhealthy for you. However, we all know that it is not the easiest thing to do. The temptation is everywhere! How can you resist on a red hot summer's day when you reach the nearest sheltered cafe, then you see at first sight a waiter serve someone an ice-cold frost bottle of Coca Cola? The droplets of water that collect on the bottle run down from the bottle rim, licking the bold red label with the familiar logo. It sends a message to your brain, which instantly craves the taste of those sugary, dark-colored fizzy bubbles. There's no doubt you wouldn't kill for a Coca Cola right now is there? It is the result of effective branding, which has undoubtedly developed with technology and media marketing over the last forty years; ever since the eighties, when they managed to eliminate fats from people's diet and lay rest the fear for sugar for a while. Then, the Bliss Point theory developed by Dr. Howard Moskowitz opened out for a whole mass of industries that poured in by the hundreds and took the formula to make their own versions of the perfect taste in a variety of different products. However, with so much competition arising in the food industry, it meant that people had to pay slowly on marketing, which they did. They also utilized the ideology of artists such as Andy Warhol in the 1950s from the Pop Art movement that played with bold colors, black and white pop-out catchphrases, and repetitive imagery to reach out to the public more effectively. The art movement that celebrated the rise of consumerism worked at inspiring a world, which is now consumed by it. When you see the phrases stand out to you every day in big, bold writing by whatever advertising medium, which is becoming more efficient with modern technology. They send you adverts backed by subliminal messages that encourage your mind to remember them. They are familiar to you, and so is the taste- of sugar. It is a difficult situation we are in, and sugar, as well as advertising, has taken hold of our minds. We are fully controlled by it, and by the system, or should I say - the infrastructure of businesses that keep it going.

Coca Cola has had such effect with its bold and bright red advertising logo that it has fashion lines run off it that make nearly as much, as the sugary drinks themselves. They have bought over companies, as have Cadbury's, which have spread their name further. Fanta, Sprite, Nestea, Schweppes are all owned under one big name. It is hard to believe that Coca Cola has such an influence on our cultural beliefs that in most countries, we associate the colors of Christmas, and especially Santa Claus, with being red and white. It all started with the popular advertisements, which were released at Christmas time with Santa Claus dressed in red and red driving a sleigh, or should I say truck full of Coca Cola through the snow. The famous chorus choir in the background sings:

"Tis the season it's always the real thing

Holidays are coming

Holidays are coming

Holidays are coming

Holidays are coming

Holidays are coming

Holidays are coming

Always Coca Cola"

How many memories does this advert bring? We indeed associate Christmas with good times, and family, and fond memories. However, we also associate it with Coca Cola, and that nostalgic advert that was always playing in the background - "Always Coca Cola!" Well, it was so compelling we now see Santa Claus dressed in red and white forever.

When companies begin to brand and advertise their products to such effect, especially when it gets into the nostalgic part of our brain, then it will have long-lasting and indefinite repercussions. We are not only addicted and reliant on the product, we are familiar with it. We cannot resist it, but we must! Remember, how many teaspoons of sugar are in a can of soft drink? It is only advertising, so switch over the channel, or pick up a book on the way home from work. Try not to let the product names bombard you, or give in to their temptation because you are stronger than you think.

4.5. SUGARY DRINKS GO ONE STEP FURTHER…

I am going to dedicate a whole chapter to what I believe to be the demons of the food sweetener industry. That is the companies that specialize in making soda or fizzy drinks, which again use sugar as their main ingredient. The reason why they are so bad is because they have one of the highest levels of concentrated sugar, generally in the form of high fructose corn syrup than any other product. They contribute to much of the health issues surrounding excessive sugar consumption. You may find this hard to believe because how could it be possible you put weight on from drinking something? You are supposed to be hydrating yourself, right? Well, you certainly are not hydrating yourself. The only liquid that will really hydrate you is water. Sometimes, by adding lemon juice, you can hydrate yourself even more. However, anything else is almost all bad for you unless freshly made. Any drink, which comes processed, whether it includes fizzy soda, fruit juice, concentrated cordial, even flavored water, is high in sugar. All these drinks include anywhere from 5-10 teaspoons of sugar in each average single serving of 330ml, which is roughly one large glass.

Therefore, imagine if you are used to consuming these drinks in high quantities, on top of sugary snacks, ready-made meals, foods that include processed foods like pizza, and pasta sauce. The list is endless, which include types of sugar, whether in it's sweetened HFCS form, or ordinary refined sugar. Now you start to realize it; you might see that you are taking in lots more sugar than you imagined. However, this is not your fault; it is what the food industries intended. They intended for you to be oblivious to that a can of soda contains ten teaspoons of sugar because you probably would not buy it. However, now you have, and you have tried it, then it is hard to kick the habit. Soda drinks are massively addictive, and they can be consumed at an exceeding rate. It is what makes them so dangerous to our health. They are the complete cognitive deception. They have high levels of sugar, which makes them addictive. Then when we drink them, we think we are hydrating ourselves, which we are not. In fact, we are de-hydrating ourselves drinking them. Therefore, we drink more, which means we are adding even more dangerously high levels of sugar to our system. Then because fructose, which is in soda drinks, shuts down the part of your brain to tell you that you are full, you will carry consuming soda till it goes out of fashion, which is never!

Brands, such as Coca Cola, spend heavily on marketing, which has encouraged the rise in its sales considerably, as well as fashion icons in the branding world. It has become one of the most widely used logos in merchandising, not just drinks, of course, but clothes, accessories, furnishings, the lot. There is nothing that Coca Cola isn't seen branded on. They have become so famous with their traditional marketing methods imprints the in most culture's beliefs. In other words, it is like we feel at home holding a bottle of Coca Cola. It is seen most effectively in their video advertising, where they created the famous Christmas advert, as well as adverts where they patent their own songs. Then they sponsor a whole list of famous people and events, such as the World Cup soccer games.

4.6. FALLING DOWN THE RABBIT HOLE

"So let us take a hop through the rabbit hole, shall we Alice?…"
Let us say we have followed the white rabbit on our search for sugar, and he takes us down a deep dark hole full of crazy mayhem. We have become crazed by the sugar rush that it feeds us. Large corporate companies have become crazed by the money it makes them. Then there are the crazy webs

of lies that have been set down to protect the industries' profits. It is slightly mad too that we were made to believe our whole diet plan is different because doctors and scientists were told to do so. Yet why were told this? The reason can be explained through the innocent tale of *Alices Adventures in Wonderland (1865),* written by the English author Lewis Carroll and then released in a cartoon movie by Disney in 1951. It was re-worked again by Tim Burton in 2010. However, all follow the same storyline where Alice meets a collection of characters in a surreal fantasy world of anthropomorphic creatures. However, the whole tale seems a little *trippy,* which has led people to believe that the story, especially the Disney production, resembles a drug trip. It is seen that some of the characters have drug addictions like the snail who is smoking a *funny* pipe, but also the Queen of hearts, who is addicted to jam tarts - or should I say sugar. What Carroll was aiming to portray was a young girl who faces a future in an industrialized world that will have to grow out of childhood into adulthood, where she will have to fend for herself. How funny is it that Carroll chose to associate his Queen of tarts with a sugar addiction? She is a crazed woman that keeps everyone under her control because of her addiction to sugar. Maybe, that is why they want to keep us under control with sugar because, in a crazed way, it makes the people on top feel in control. Therefore, they control us with their magic white ingredient - sugar. Most of us are not aware of it. I would imagine that most of you were not aware of half the facts I have shared with you so far. We are blind to most of what goes on under the network because we are too busy with our everyday world and daily pressures. A great many of us lead stressful lives at work or home, so we do not pick up on the warning signs. Instead, we indulge in a sweet snack now and then to overcome the pressure a little. It rewards us, so we find ourselves dipping into a bag of crisps, opening a chocolate bar, or taking a sip of sweet soft drink. The instant buzz it gives us tides us over, although, with time, we find that we crave more. We then look for it as a comfort, especially if our circumstances in life become a little more stressful. So we eat more sugar. Then as we get older or the workload gets higher - we have less time to exercise.

That is when you start to go down the dark and bumpy black hole, you begin to pick up pace, and the effects get a little worse, and faster as you eat more. Before you know it, you are in your mid-forties slightly overweight and on the verge of Diabetes 2. You are lost down the burrow with temptation fed to in heavy advertising, and a lack of awareness. We do not know how much sugar is in that product that we are marketed over and over again. We also do not understand why the system chose to lie to us for so many decades. We just followed the signs, and the messages that were fed to us on the way, those that said - EAT ME on it, in big, bold letters. It might change our shape completely and adversely for the worst, yet we are unaware of it because we are instructed to eat it. That is what the system did. They told us to eat sugar, and that is what we did. However, it is why, as Dr. Robert Ludwig proclaimed passionately to us in 2009, "we are all getting sick!"

5

Toxic Sugar

Sugar is toxic; there is no doubt about it! We were lied to for decades and told to eat less saturated fats by scientists and nutritionists, such as Ancel Keys, because allegedly cholesterol is linked to heart disease. Well, it is not; it is good for the heart. Not only were we lied to, but we were told the absolute opposite. We were told to take out an ingredient that our heart needs, and said to replace it with something it doesn't need. What is worse is it will do long-lasting damage to our heart, and will essentially result in heart disease. We have looked at why they might have decided to provide us with this false information, and now we are going to look at what it has done to us. We saw before in chapter 3.3. *Sugar In Our Body- Glucose,* when we eat sugar in excess, whether it is fructose, but especially sucrose, then our blood sugar levels go up. As our body already produces its own sugar in glucose, then excess sugar that we ingest harms our sugar-making machine, which is the liver.

The liver will turn the glucose into body fuel, which is glycerol, and then stored in body cells and muscle mass with the lip of your pancreas secreting insulin. However, insulin, which controls the blood sugar levels to bring it down to a steady rate, also only expects a certain amount of sugar in the blood. It has a biological clock that has developed over hundreds of thousands of years, which has never taken in so much sugar. Therefore, it finds it hard to control the levels after so long. That is where you start to see the current issues, which is a rising pandemic of people suffering, or who are expected to suffer from Diabetes type 2. It is an illness like obesity, where we store too much body fat in glucose and fatty acids excreted from carbohydrates, as well as our dental hygiene, which is at risk - cavities, tooth decay, etc. Then when you imagine that your liver can only take so much strain from the work you are giving it with the sugar, you are over-feeding it all the time—liver disease, as well as liver failure, dialysis, etc. Then, of course, there are the effects that the sugar levels, as well as the addictive dependency, have on your temperament and mood swings. It has also been associated with Alzheimer's disease that could be another side-effect to the effect of excess sugar on our blood sugar levels. Unfortunately, as a result of what we were recommended, then these health issues have soared out of control. I am going to share with you in this chapter just how dangerous sugar can be too our diet. We are living in a toxic modern world where sugar is a wanted culprit for the temptation it gives us. When the craving becomes a habit, it also becomes a compulsive disorder that controls us. It is not only the mind, which is regulated, but the body is too. It is like a ticking time bomb waiting to give in when it has taken too much sugar.

5.1. DENTAL HYGIENE

So when did the first dentists arrive on the scene?...
The pioneer to dentistry was Pierre Fauchard (1678-1761), who was a French Physician and published the book *Le Chirurgien Dentiste* ("The Surgeon Dentist") in 1728. However, the dentistry schooling did not become widespread until the 19th century. In 1828 the first dental school opened up in Bainbridge, Ohio, where many of the first dentists studied and made their career. Then in 1840, the first dental college opened in Baltimore, Maryland, in the US called Baltimore College of Dental Surgery. It was at the same time that sugar production was booming in America, and people were beginning to get a taste for its *pleasurable* taste. However, very few people could afford dental care in the 1800s, and often settled for a nasty trip to the barbers, or blacksmith's who would take 'tooth extraction' up as a part-time job. It is widely known that sugar is directly connected to tooth decay. Therefore, if we did not eat sugar, we would not need dentists.

Unfortunately, sugar is so toxic to our teeth, and it can damage them very quickly. Therefore, if you do not want to find yourself sifting through a whole pile of dental and medical bills, then you should take more care of your teeth.

After we consume foods with sugar, whether in small doses or large, the fructose molecules combine with our saliva and bacteria, which is in our mouth to help break down the food. It is highly acidic and will instantly attack and work at dissolving the enamel on your teeth. These attacks usually last around twenty minutes until it completely disappears from your saliva. Therefore, if you regularly snack out on sugary foods or drinks, then you are continually exposing your teeth to acidic attacks, which are slowly but surely attacking your teeth. Sugary beverages have high concentrations of sugar and are one of the worse things for your teeth. Anything from juice to energy drinks and flavored water, sweets, and even milk in large quantities will work at eroding your teeth away because it contains lactose, which is a natural made sugar.

Over time, the regular loss of enamel will lead to tooth cavities and a build of plaque in and around the teeth and gums. Cavities are permanently damaged areas to the hard surface or enamel of your teeth, where the plaque has eaten away at it. Your teeth start to rot away, and small holes begin to appear that over time worsen and break the tooth. Teeth will become sensitive, and often very painful. Toothache has been described as one of the torturous pains you can experience in your life, which is normally your nerve sensors telling you that the cavities have caused infection in the gums, and it is time to remove your tooth.

It is advised for most people who have poor dental hygiene, or a build-up of plaque to follow these health tips:

1) Eat less sugar
2) Snack on sugary snacks less regularly, leaving a few hours in between
3) Always wash your mouth out with water when you eat or drink acidic, sugary products
4) Brush your teeth 30 minutes after snacking on sugary items
5) Fluoride treatment (an intense clean at the dentists now and again)

6)   Chew sugarless gum - Xylitol is especially suitable for reducing cavity-reducing bacteria

7)   Neutralize acidity in your mouth with elevated pH mouthwash

So, there you have it, folks! If you want to save those ultra-expensive dentist bills, cut down on the sugar. When you start to look at, sugar is one deadly money-making commodity that not only controls us, but slowly destroys. We would save so much money, so much pain and hardship if we did not consume so much sugar. It might be a 'guilty pleasure,' we find it hard to resist. However, when you start to see the real picture, and just how destructive it can be to your teeth, your body and your mind; maybe you would be willing to take the risk to resist it. You do not have to cut it out altogether, just limit it considerably. Make sure that you allow yourself limited 'sweet treats,' save them for exceptional moments. You will love them all the more! Learn to get control over your snack times, and your teeth will stay gleaming white for years to come, and no empty pockets.

5.2. DIABETES PANDEMIC

Diabetes, also known as *diabetes mellitus,* is a human-made disease, which was first recorded in the Egyptian times, and also documented by the famous Egyptian physicist Hey-Ra. He noted that frequent urination was a symptom of some unknown disease, which also caused emaciation. Then the word itself derives from the Greek word diabetes and the Latin word *mellitus,* which means 'honeyed or sweet.' The Ancient Romans and Greeks saw that the disease correlated with finding too much sugar in the blood and urine. Finally, it was not until 1889, when Joseph Von Mering and Oscar Minkowski became credited with the role of diagnosing the first case of diabetes, as an illness that was an effect of imbalanced blood sugar levels caused in the pancreas. In other words, when your pancreas is unable to produce enough insulin, or is insulin resistant. Remember that we secrete insulin to calm down our blood sugar levels in the process of glycogenolysis, which is where we store glycerol in our body, and if it cannot be stored in muscle mass or the liver, then it gets stored as body fat. In 1936 a British scientist called Harold Percival Himsworth differentiated two types of diabetes called Diabetes type-1 and type-2. Scientists believe that Diabetes type 1 is a genetic disease or possibly a side-effect caused by environmental factors like viruses. In this case, the DNA of your body is adversely set in self-destruct mode. In other words, your self-defense mechanisms, instead of fighting infection, will attack and destroy the insulin-producing beta cells that are trying to work in the pancreas. Diabetes type-2, on the other hand, is self-inflicted. It is a chronic disease that develops until your body is unable to produce enough insulin to maintain your blood sugar levels, or your body becomes resilient to it instead. When this happens, your blood sugar levels either become dangerously high or low. The body can no longer work like it should; it can longer work the process of glycogenolysis. Therefore, instead of moving the glycerol into your cells, it will move it into your bloodstream. As blood sugar levels increase, then the insulin-producing beta cells release even more insulin, until they eventually become impaired and produce none. You can usually diagnose the moment when the insulin beta cells are over-powering your bloodstream before they damage themselves as pre-diabetes. Therefore, people are given the warning signs before it is too late.

Even still, Diabetes type 2 is massively on the rise. Although it is not directly, Diabetes type-2 is not directly caused by the toxic effects of sugar. It is linked to people becoming overweight because of eating too much sugar, which is when the insulin beta cells become damaged. When Diabetes type 2 is left untreated, or becomes chronic, then it will become life-threatening. It is what keeps the fuel in your body moving, if this mechanism of producing insulin is disabled, then so does your body stop working, and your organs will start to break-down. It is like a car with a faulty engine that cannot burn the fuel properly to move forward. Diabetes increases the risk of the following health issues to arise:

1) Heart diseases
2) High blood pressure
3) Stroke

4)   Atherosclerosis (thinning of the blood vessels)

5)   Nerve damage - loss of feeling the limbs (causes nausea, diarrhea, constipation and erectile dysfunction)

6)   Amputation of the legs or feet

7)   Kidney Disease

8)   Eye damage (cataracts, glaucoma, blindness, etc.)

9)   Slow healing of wounds with higher risks of infection

10)   Hearing impairments

11)   Skin conditions including bacterial and fungal infections

12)   Sleep apnea, which can lead to further health issues

13)   Alzheimer's disease

14)   Liver disease

15)   Cancer

The list seems endless; does it not?…

You could link nearly every common illness and health deficiency to Diabetes. Unfortunately, over the last 50 years, due to the damage that was made to the modern health system by scientists, such as Ancel Keys and the three Harvard graduate from 1967, who said that saturated fats caused heart disease. However, as I said before, it is not. Instead, it is good for the heart, especially Omega 3 fatty acids found in fish oil. However, instead of eating correctly, we have been poisoning ourselves collectively with sugar. When your body reaches a stage that is at the risk of Diabetes type 2, it is your body telling you: "Stop! Do not feed me any more sugar because I cannot process it." That is why most older people suffer from it. They have exposed themselves to sugar for so many decades. Then as they get older, their organs become less resilient, which is when they have a higher chance of developing Diabetes type 2. However, the 21st century has seen a horrific rise in cases of Diabetes 2 in children that are overweight. We are not just affecting ourselves with excessive sugar, but we are putting our children in danger too. They are innocent to the fact that sugar is harmful, and they are also very attracted to its sweet taste. Often, parents will give in and feed their children all the sugar they ask for, especially if they suffer from a sugar addiction, and obesity themselves. How many families do you see where the children are just as overweight as their parents? It is extremely dangerous for a child whose digestive system and body is still developing. Imagine if you damage the whole system, when it hasn't even finished growing? Well, the results are catastrophic and also very sad because kids are not in control at all. They rely on the correct conditioning, which is to eat as much sugar as possible, and live a 'short and unhealthy' life. We are still being taught the opposite of how to live correctly.

Today diabetes has reached a pandemic state where 422 million people suffer from its worldwide. That is more than the entire population of the United States. In 2035, it is expected to reach 600 million cases of Diabetes. Therefore, a change has to be made quick to reverse the effects what the *World Health Organization* projects to happen. Equally, obesity is spiraling even further out of control. Six years ago, in 2014, it was recorded that 1.3 billion people were overweight - that is the population of China. However, in 2025, which is in just five years, the expected rate of obesity is expected to reach 2.9 million people. That is a third of the worldwide population. That is why I mentioned before, for so many millennia, we stood as the Homo sapiens. Sapiens raised on two legs in a normal erect stature of average weight. However, in the last forty years, we have seen a new shaped-man altogether, one that could change our prehistoric shape forever.

5.3. OBESITY OUT OF CONTROL

Now, as we have seen, the numbers of cases rise in Diabetes 2 considerably, so we have also seen obesity rise even more. The two illnesses are directly linked. As we have discussed when the amount of sugar in your system is higher than your cells and liver can store, then your liver turns it into body fat, which you keep building up if you do not burn it off. That is when you are at the risk of putting on more weight because your body will keep storing it an unlimited rate. As the brain works in reverse to what your body wants it to do at times. In other words, the reward part of your mind will crave more sugar; until it reaches a stage it wants an unlimited supply of it. It is possible, as fructose dangerously, shuts down the part of your brain that says you are full. In other words, you can keep eating sugar at an unlimited rate, but we will only store it as body fat. Sugar is all calories and no nutrients; it will do nothing but produce toxic waste in your system- body fat!

People have different metabolic rates. Therefore, some people burn off more energy and fat than others. People that have a slower metabolism have the risk of putting on more weight faster. Slow metabolism is often caused by people that try to lose weight in the wrong ways. In other words, if people follow low-calorie diets, which are low in fat, but high in sugar, then they effectively damage their metabolism and slow it down. A low-calorie diet is what we are told to follow when we are overweight. However, it is again false information, which reverses how our process of metabolism works. We are over-stressing our body! It was proven in a reality tv program called *The Biggest Loser,* which was aired for the first time in the U.S. in 2004. In the program, contestants who suffered severely with obesity were told to follow a low-calorie diet plan, as well as carry out intensive physical exercise and activities to attempt to lose pounds of weight, dangerously fast - they over-stressed their body and metabolic rate. Weight loss should be carried out properly, following the right diet, and not necessarily cutting out calories, but eating the right things that produce those calories. We will look at this in more detail in the next chapter, but also remember section *2.2. Counting Calories.*

In 2015, an American scientist called Kevin Hall was skeptical at the dieting regime the contestants were told to follow. Therefore, he decided to carry out a follow-up investigation of the contestants that took part in the series that was aired in 2009. Not only had he noticed that all the contestants, including the winner, had gained weight again, he also noted that they had damaged their metabolic rate. It made it harder for them to lose weight afterward.

One such contestant, named Danny Cahill weighed 426 pounds when he started the program in 2009. Over just seven months, he lost the equivalent of 236 pounds, resulting in his final weight at the end of the program resting at 190 pounds. Six years later, he had gained 101 pounds, which meant that he had gone back up to weighing 291 pounds. However, what was more shocking was that it had damaged his metabolism so severely, that it worked at 800 calories slower than a person of his weight should burn off. This same effect had happened to all the other 14 contestants. Therefore, obesity is not just on the rise. It is very difficult to break out of because doctors and dieticians are not giving the right advice on how people should go about losing weight.

5.4. MENTAL HEALTH AND ALZHEIMER'S DISEASE

Sugar and living on a high-carb diet has been implicated in the progression of mental decline and dementia with time. A person with high blood sugar levels or diabetes can be shown to cause memory problems that are linked to Alzheimer's disease. As it is known that diabetes can weaken a person's blood vessels, then not only will it increase the risk of various types of dementia, and also the onset of a stroke. It has been linked to the insulin resistance that is suffered by people with diabetes. As the sugar cannot enter the body cells, not even in the brain, then slowly like all the other organs, it will begin to breakdown, and cognitive activity will decline.

On the other hand, guess what can reverse the effects of dementia and also increase your brain activity?

 That's right - saturated fats! Now, are you beginning to see the severity of the lies, which we were told in the 1970s and 80s? I can imagine you feel very deceived. However, now you know the truth, you also know that you are in control. Your mind is not controlled by sugar. You are in control of your mind, and you can actively limit the amount of sugar you eat. You might have some side-effects to start. They can last anywhere from a few days to 2 - 3 weeks. However, this depends on your dependency and the severity of your sugar addiction. The withdrawal symptoms you are likely to expect include:

1) Depression
2) Anxiety
3) Restlessness
4) Tiredness
5) Lack of concentration
6) Dizziness
7) Irritability
8) Mood swings- anger
9) Nausea

Have you noticed how all these health issues are almost all directed to the mind? Therefore, it is not your body that cries for sugar; it is your mind. Although it is difficult to get passed these withdrawal symptoms, they soon start to fade away, and you will have fewer cravings for sugar. Even when you see it, it will be less tempting because you haven't got excess sugar in your system, but also you have trained your brain to stop asking you for sugar. Sometimes, we have to take a step back and mentally condition ourselves when issues, especially addictions to substances like sugar, take over our minds. Well, we have to get back control. When people suffer from harmful habits to sugar, which then has a life-threatening effect on their health, then it is important to seek someone who can help you condition your mind back to basics. Those basics are your survival mode, which is at the moment programmed in self-destruction mode because your mind has lost control of itself. It could be due to other personal issues, which is why you seek out the reward of a sugary treat to make yourself feel better. However, this sort of escapism is short-lived and more destructive to our physical and mental health in the long run. There are plenty of ways to escape, which are more constructive and promote a healthier way of living.

6
What's next?

So there you have it, the real truth about sugar! And what happens next? Do you think it is time to sit back, relax, and watch the world go by? Or do you think it is time to make a change? Well, what will happen if we decide not to? It is much easier to ignore the issues at hand, and pretend like nothing is wrong. However, the numbers are real, and they also keep rising. It could be that in fifteen years, and then a third of the world population is obese. However, at the rate that these numbers are rising, which is super-fast, so imagine in fifty years' time. The way the numbers are looking, and especially in the United States, which has the highest rate of obesity in the world. It would mean that roughly 95% of Americans are expected to be overweight in 2050. Therefore, are you ready to make a change? Unfortunately, we have seen that everything we are told is not always right. In fact, we were told for decades that we should not eat saturated fats, so that the fault could be taken away from sugar and carbohydrates. However, this had reverse effects because sugar is toxic, and saturated fats help us do everything that sugar does not. Sugar destroys us. We were advised to destroy ourselves, not live healthily. However, now we know the truth, and we know not to believe the doctors, or the media, or see past the advertising, which is only set there to control and tempt you with more sugar. It is time that you took control of your own life so that you can foresee your future retirement happy and healthy, rather than in and out of hospital. It is up to you, so no need to point the finger at anyone. Take the information you have learned here and spread the word! You never know you might just save one more human life, as well as the divine body shape we were born with. You only get one, so feed it with the right things, and don't always give in to your mental desires.

6.1. DON'T BELIEVE EVERYTHING THE DOCTOR SAYS

Now, the information I want to share must be taken lightly because we will all need a trip to the doctors at some point in our life. Our health system, which includes all the doctors and nurses, work hard every day to save thousands of lives, which they do very well! Without doctors and nurses, many of us would not have the chance in life that we do. Therefore, I am in no way condemning their work. They work hard in giving excellent counsel to patients with conditions such as obesity and diabetes. They are also told to follow a specific protocol. It governs all the advice and information they give about tackling weight problems, and possibly avoiding or reversing the effect of diabetes, amongst other health issues. However, this protocol comes from higher up. It comes from the Institutions and the government. Therefore, as in the 70s and 80s, these three entities are linked. However, when you start to look at who funds who, then you see that, sometimes not all the information we are given is set to help us. For example, consider who pays for the doctor's bills - we do! Who keeps the doctors in business by getting sick? That's right - we do! So, take a look at Robert Lustig's heartfelt proclamation that "when fat went down, sugar went up, and we're all getting sick." Do you start to see the full picture now? It is all a money-making business that needs business to generate business, which, if it means taking lives at risk and changing the future world for the worst, then so be it! It is the world we are moving into, one that is not controlled by people anymore but entities - big corporate companies. However, the trouble is these entities are not people; they are fictive beings. Therefore, they have no empathy, and hold no responsibility, or guilt for the unfortunate future, which we are in for if we do not make the change ourselves.

6.2. DON'T COUNT CALORIES

Once upon a time, they gave us bad advice, which led to the pandemic we are in today and seen most severely in cases of obesity and diabetes. They also continue to supply us false advice to protect the fact that they gave us bad advice in the first place. Therefore, we have been fed lies on top of lies. One such false theory was one that we should worry about, which is when we started counting calories. We are told to eat low-calorie diets so that we can lose weight. We are also advised to look at the back of the food packages because it will tell us how many calories are in the dish, and if it is high in calories, then we should not eat it.

Do you believe this? If you do, then like everyone, you believe another lie to the system. We have been known to associate calories with food, since 1887 when the American chemist, Wilbur Olin Atwater, carried out an experiment where he burnt different food groups like carbohydrates, fats, etc. to see how many calories they generated. He discovered that fat produced nine calories as opposed to four calories in carbs. From this theory, the American writer, Lulu Hunt Peters, decided to publish one of the first books in dieting in 1918, called *Diet and Health (with the keys to calories)*. She theorized from Atwater's theory that calories were linked to weight gain. Her theory proposed that the more calories you eat, the more calories you had to burn.

This theory became used by most dieticians, until our modern-day society regards weight gain with calories. We are told to eat an average of 1500-2000 calories a day, and if we eat anymore, then we will have to burn that extra amount off, or it will be stored as excess fat. Does this sound familiar to you? However, the basis of this theory, which Atwater discovered again, is slightly, if not very, inaccurate. It is because he did not distinguish each food group well enough. He wrote down his results, yet never considered that even though fats have more calories, which they do, we also burn them off a lot quicker too. We do this for a reason, and that is because saturated fats are a more healthy fuel for us to burn, so we burn it quicker. The trouble in the 20th century is that all the information on dietary and nutritional advice decided to favor the two theories made by Lulu Hunt Peters and Ancel Keys. Their conclusions lacked reliable evidence because there was no other information on the contrary. There was only Yudkin's argument, which was not voiced because he was not as famous or influential, as Keys was in the 1970s.

However, it was not just a mere mistake they made, was it?... It was pretty grave on the scheme of things!

6.3 LEARN TO READ THE LABELS

Now you know the truth; it is time to take a better look at the labels. In other words, we need to stay away from the low-fat options because of their deceiving. Fat is not the issue - sugar is. When you are next in the supermarket, and you see the low-fat options and compare them with the ordinary fat, take mayonnaise, and see if the sugar levels are any different. When you see that the sugar levels are the same, then you know that this is a deceiving product. The chances are if you buy it, you will put more weight on, as well as risk your health more, than if you buy the ordinary fat options.

Another way food industries lie to us is with their food labels. They use names and metric measurements of nutrition and different ingredients, so that we cannot understand them. They are made for a professional to read who has studied this information. Most of us do not know all the different names they use for sugar. We also not realize that they have downsized the metric unit of sugar to every 100g so that it appears to be less than it is. In other words, if a tin of food contains 250g but the ingredients read per 100g, then the amount of sugar in it is going to be more than double. However, we are not programmed to make that calculation because we merely read what is printed on the label.

Food labels are the last hope for the food industry now. Therefore, they will deceive us with the information they print on it, as much as possible. However, it only takes some awareness, as well as time and patience, reading the labels to check what it is you are actually eating. Make sure it is healthy and good for you, and that it is not high in sugar or carbohydrates. Find out all the names they use for sugar, if you are not sure of any ingredients on the food label, and then search it. You can easily access Google search these days on your mobile device. Make sure you keep on top of your diet from on. You might not be showing any health factors just yet, but every day you eat healthier, and then you add another day to your life. You also eliminate an extra day in the hospital when your body starts to show any irreversible, negative signs of eating too much sugar.

www.ingramcontent.com/pod-product-compliance
Lightning Source LLC
Chambersburg PA
CBHW051219250726
48655CB00006B/2494